The Little Yellow book Of Medical Mnemonics

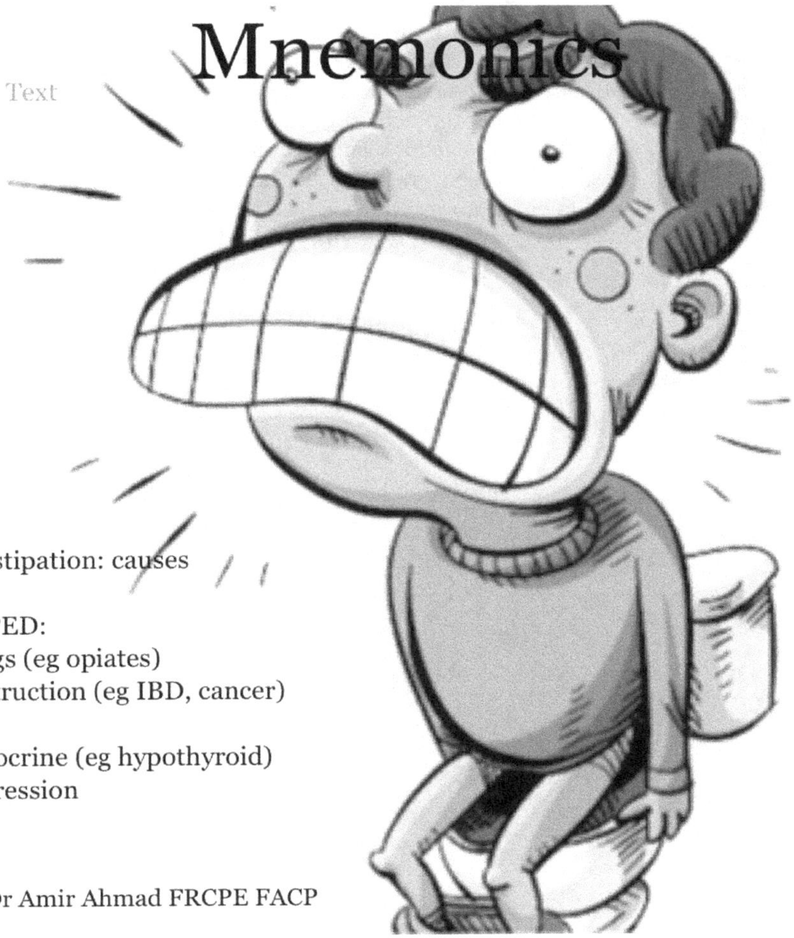

Constipation: causes

DOPED:
Drugs (eg opiates)
Obstruction (eg IBD, cancer)
Pain
Endocrine (eg hypothyroid)
Depression

Dr Amir Ahmad FRCPE FACP

Preface

Medicine is a vast subject often requiring large amounts of information to be remembered which is challenging. Mnemonics can be very helpful if they are good and relate to the topic that needs memorising. This book mainly focuses on those mnemonics which relate to topics commonly encountered in frontline Medicine rather than in exams. So it avoids theoretical topics like features of Fedreich's ataxia which is rarely seen in clinical practice by GPs or Acute Medics and is seen in exams only. Rather it covers topics like causes of Pneumothorax which is seen in everyday practice. I hope you will find the book useful.

Dr Amir Ahmad
July 2020

Published from UK. All rights reserved
Copyright Dr Amir Ahmad

Acknowledgement

I thank everyone who have been kind enough to provide some of the Mnemonics used.

Contents

. Headache - hyperkalemia- page 1- 10

. Urinary incontinence- vomiting-page 11-20

. Stroke - abdominal distension- 21-30

. Leukemia- pericarditis- 31-40

. ECG - asthma- 41-50

. RLQ pain - normal anion gap acidosis- 51- 60

. MYocardial infarction- san farancisco syncope - 61-70

. Massive splenomegaly - Papilloedema- 71-80

. Ptosis- morphine - 81-90

. Hepatomegaly - sensory ataxia- 91-100

. Sixth nerve palsy - hepatosplenomegaly- 101- 110

. GI obstruction- empyema -111- 120

. Haemoptysis- monoarththris - 121- 125

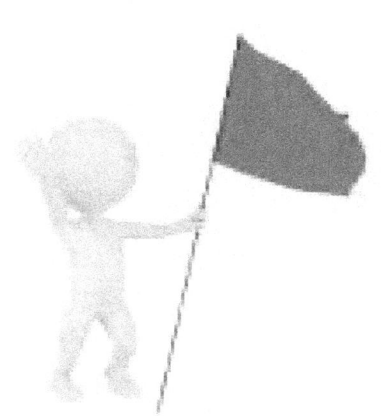

Red Flags in headache

Mnemonic: SNOOP

. Systemic signs and disorders
. Neurologic symptoms
. Onset new or changed & patient > 50 years old
. Onset in thunderclap presentation
. Papilloedema, pulsatile tinnitus. Precipitated by excercise, positional provocation

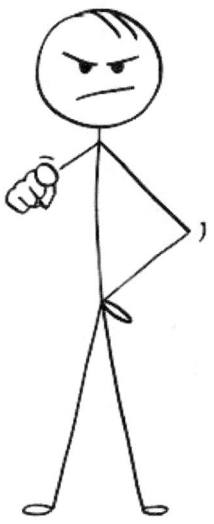

Back pain : red flag symptoms

Mnemonic: TUNA FISH

. Trauma
. Unexplained weight Loss
. Neurological symptoms
. Age > 50 years
. Fever
. IVDU
. Steroid use
. History of cancer

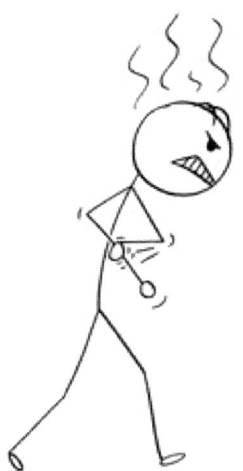

Life-Threatening Causes of Chest Pain

Mnemonic: DEATH

Dissection (aneurysm)
Embolism (pulmonary)
Acute coronary syndrome
Tension PTX
Hole in GI tract (Esophageal rupture, Perforated ulcer)

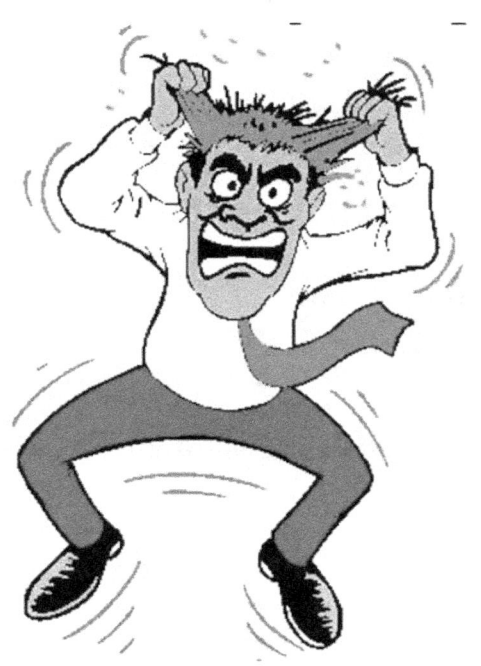

Dyspepsia symptoms

Mnemonic: ALARM

Anaemia (iron deficiency)
Loss of weight
Anorexia
Recent onset of progressive symptoms
Melaena / haematemesis
Swallowing difficulty

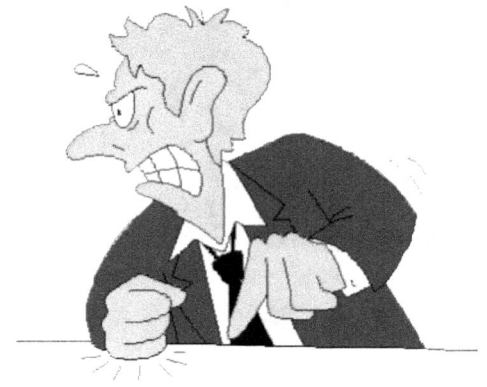

Vertigo

Mnemonic: VOMITS

. Vestibulitis
. Ototoxic drugs
. Meineire Disease
. Injury
. Tumour
. Spin (benign positional vertigo)

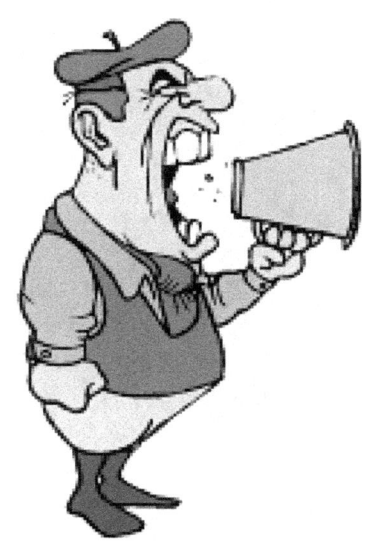

Haemoptysis : causes

. Haemorrhagic diathesis
. Edema
. Malignancy
. Others
. Pulmonary vascular abnormalities
. Trauma
. Your treatment (anticoagulation)
. SLE
. Infarction of Lungs
. Septic

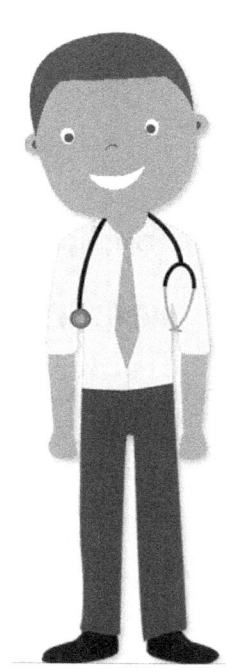

Parkinson disease: symptoms

Mnemonic: PQRST

. Paucity of expresion
. parQinson
. Rigidity
. Stooped posture
. Tremor at rest

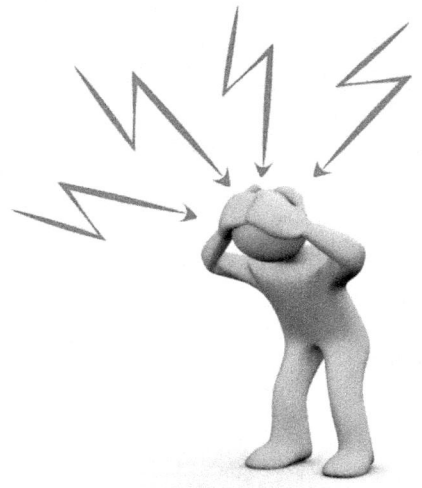

Hypernatremia

Mnemonic: MODEL

. Medications
. Osmotic diuretics
. Diabetes Insipidus
. Excessive Water
. Low water intake

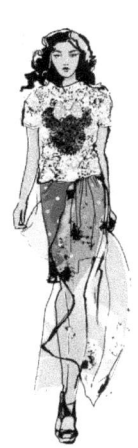

Headache Dangerous differential

Mnemonic: SIT 4 C

. Subarachnoid haemorrhage
. Intraerebral haemorrhage
. Temporal arteritis
. CNS infections.
. Carbon monoxide toxicity
. Cervical artery dissection
. Cerebral venoussinus thrombosis

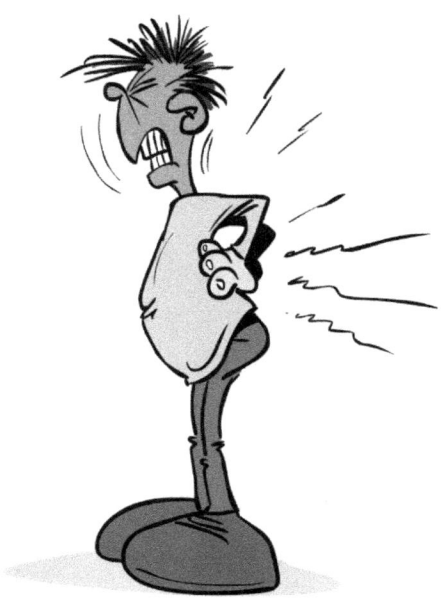

Hyperkalemia: causes

Mnemonic: MACHINE

. Medications
. Acidosis
. Cellular destruction
. Hypoaldosteronism, hemolysis
. Intake- impaired
. Nephrons, renal failure
. Excretion -impaired

The hyperkalemia machine

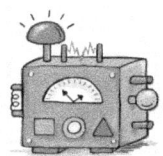

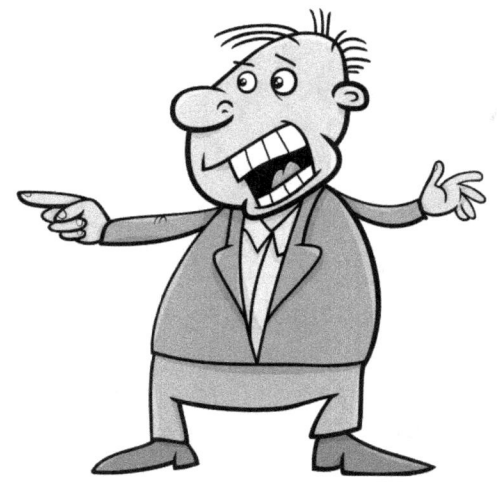

Urinarry Incontinence: causes

Mnemonic: DIAPERS

Delirium
Infection
Atrophic Urethritis
Pharmaceuticals
Psychologic
Excess Urine Output
Restricted Mobility
Stool Impaction

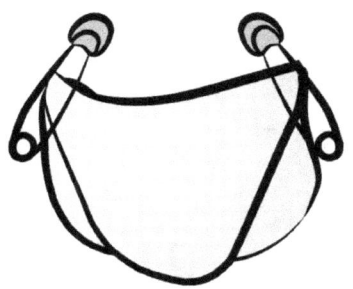

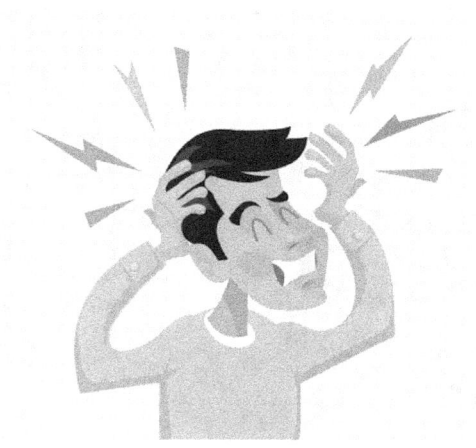

Delerium causes

Mnemonic:DELERIUM

. Drugs
. Epilepsy /electctrolyte imbalance
. Liver failure
. Infection
. Retention
. Intracranial
. Uremia
. Metabolism

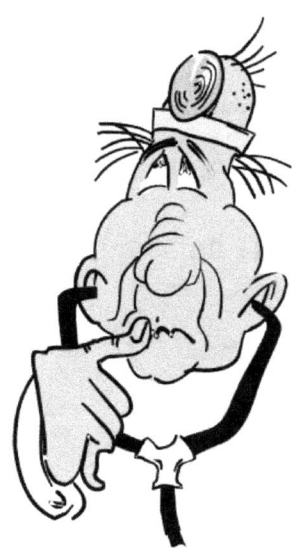

5 P's OF CIRCULATORY CHECKS

- P Pain
- P Paresthesia
- P Paralysis
- P Pulse
- P Pallor

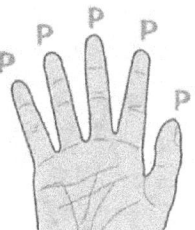

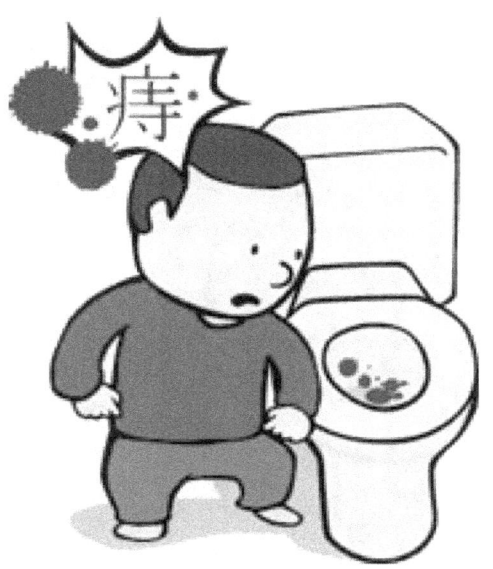

Haematuria causes

Mnemonic: HAMATURIAS

. Haemorrhagic diseases
. Endocarditis
. Malignant hypertension
. Acute Glomerulonephritis
. Tuberculosis (kidney)/Tumors (bladder)
. Urinary tract infection
. Renal infarction
. Idiopathic
. Anticoagulants
. Stones in urinary tract

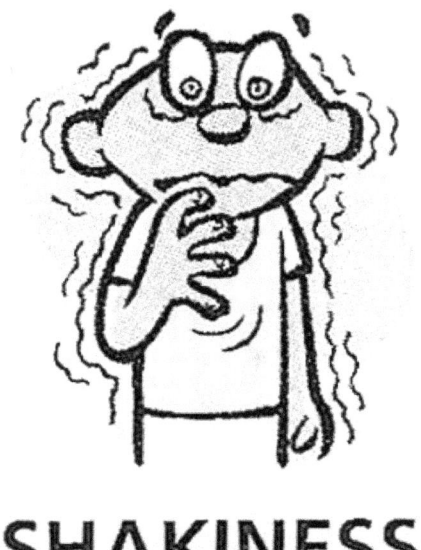

SHAKINESS

Causes of life -threatening chest pain

Mnemonic:PET-MAC

P = Pulmonary embolism
E = Esophageal rupture
T = Tension pneumothorax
M = Myocardial infarction
A = Aortic dissection
C = Cardiac tamponade

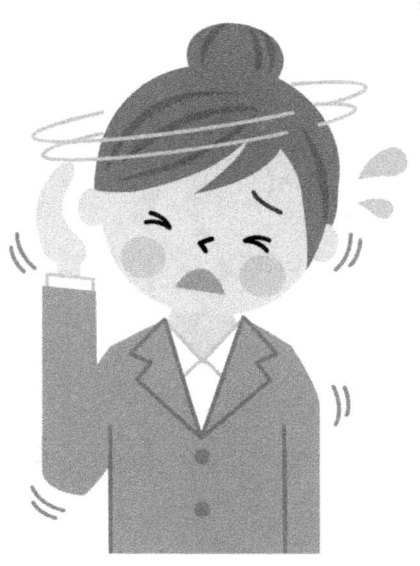

Atrial fibrillation: causes of new onset

Mnemonic: THE ATRIAL FIBS:

Thyroid
Hypothermia
Embolism (P.E.)

Alcohol
Trauma (cardiac contusion)
Recent surgery (post CABG)
Ischemia
Atrial enlargement
Lone or idiopathic

Fever, anemia, high-output states
Infarct
Bad valves (mitral stenosis)
Stimulants (cocaine, theo, amphet, caffeine)

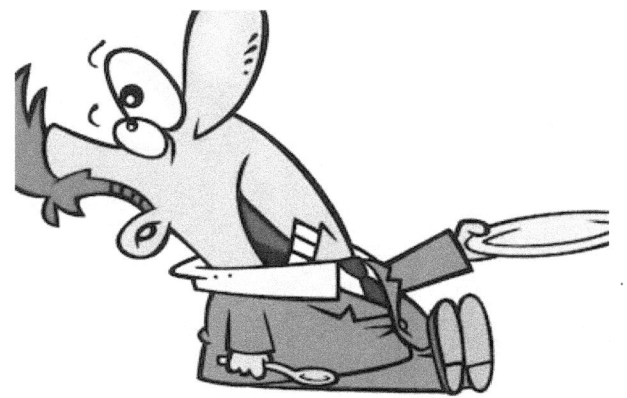

PEA/Asystole : causes

Mnemonic:ITCHPAD

Infarction

Tension pneumothorax

Cardiac tamponade

Hypovolemia/Hypothermia/Hypo-,Hyperkalemia/Hypomagnesmia/Hypoxemia

Pulmonary embolism

Acidosis

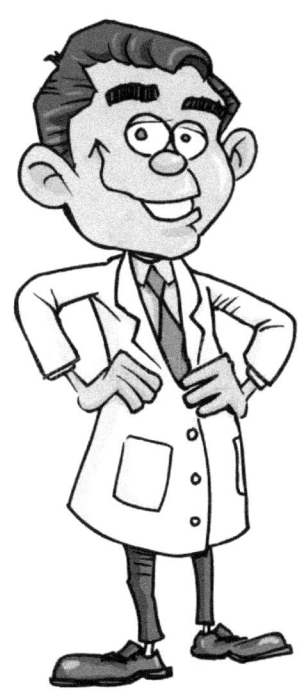

Subarachnoid haemorrhage

Mnemonic:BATS

Berry aneurysm

Arteriovenous malformation/Adult polycystic kidney disease

Trauma

Stroke

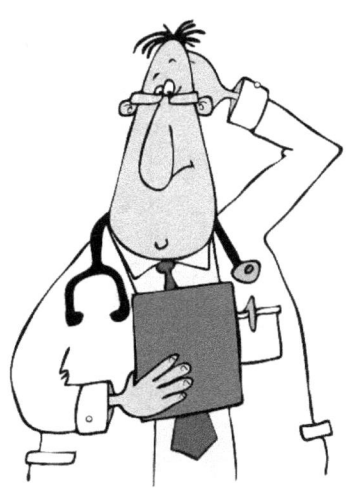

Tension Pneumothorax: signs and symptoms

Mnemonic: P-THORAX

Pleuritic pain

Tracheal deviation

Hyperresonance

Onset sudden

Reduced breath sounds (and dyspnea)

Absent fremitus

X-ray shows collapse

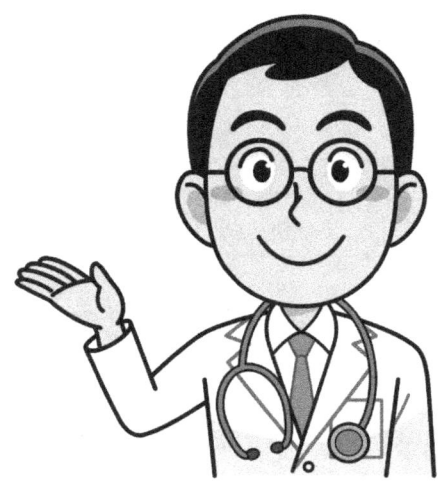

Vomiting: Non-GIT differetial

Mnemonic:ABCDEFGHI

Acute renal failure

Brain [increased ICP]

Cardiac [inferior MI]

DKA

Ears [labyrinthitis]

Foreign substances [paracetamol, theo, etc.]

Glaucoma

Hyperemesis gravidarum

Infection [pyelonephritis, meningitis]

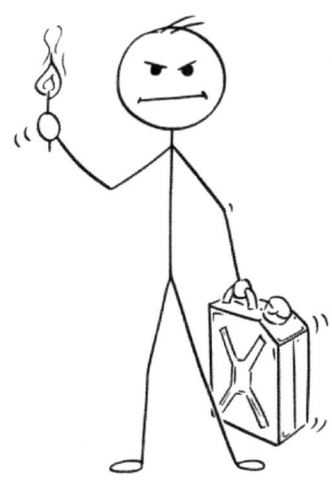

Stroke risk factors

Mnemonic:HEADS

Hypertension/ Hyperlipidemia

Elderly

Atrial fib

Diabetes mellitus/ Drugs (cocaine)

Smoking/Sex (male)

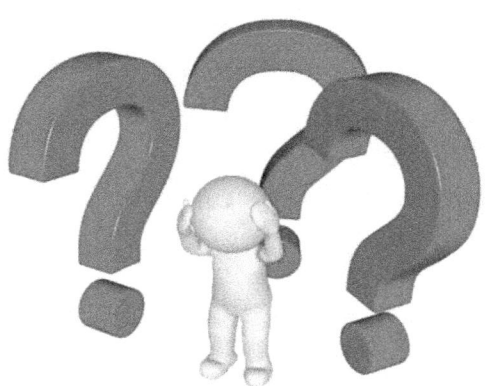

Causes of Pinpoint pupils

Pinpoint Pupils are caused by oPioids
and Pontine Pathology

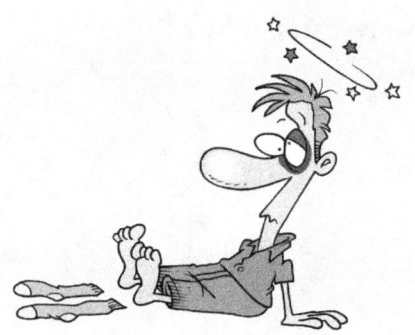

Features of a life-threatening asthma attack

Mnemonic: A CHEST

Arrhythmia/Altered conscious level
Cyanosis, PaCO2 normal
Hypotension, Hypoxia (PaO2<8kPa, SpO2 <92%)
Exhaustion
Silent chest
Threatening PEF < 33% best or predicted (in those >5yrs old)

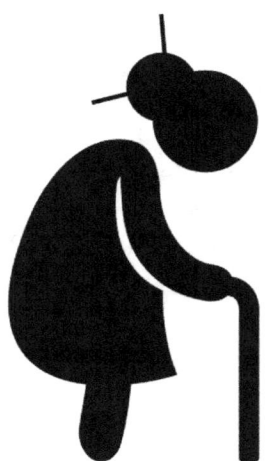

Features of normal pressure hydrocephalus

Mnemonic: Wet, Wobbly, Wacky

Wet = urinary incontinence
Wobbly = ataxic gait
Wacky = dementia

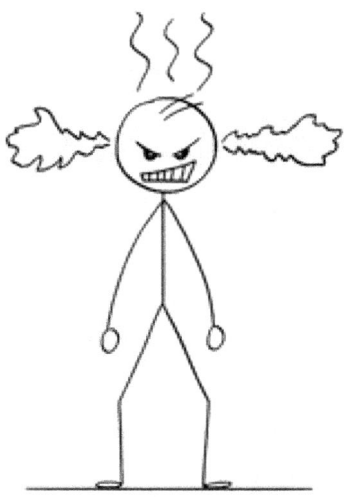

DKA precipitants (5 I's)

Infection
Ischaemia (cardiac, mesenteric)
Infarction
Ignorance (poor control)
Intoxication (alcohol)

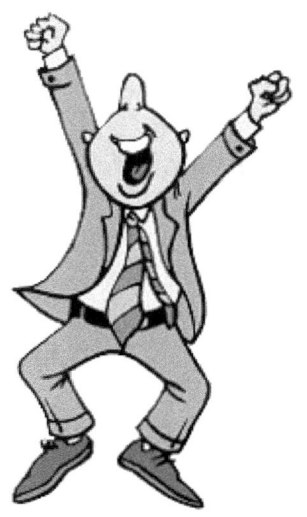

Pancreatitis causes

I GET SMASHED

Idiopathitic

Gallstones
Ethanol
Trauma

Steroids
Mumps
Autoimmune (PAN)
Scorpion stings
Hyperlipidemia/ Hypercalcemia
ERCP
Drugs

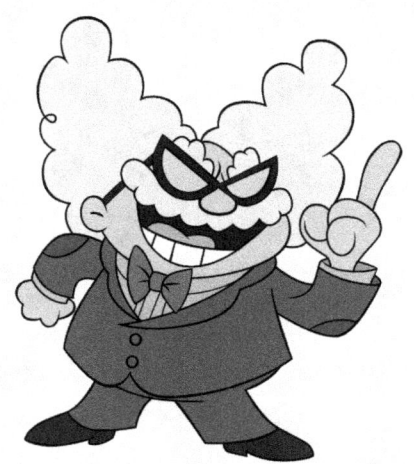

Hypercalcemia causes

CHIMPANZEES

Calcium supplementation
Hyperparathyroidism
Iatrogenic, immobilization
Multiple myeloma, milk-alkali syndrome, medication (e.g Lithium)
Parathyroid hyperplasia or adenoma
Alcohol
Neoplasm (e.g breast cancer, lung cancer)
Zollinger Ellison syndrome
Excessive Vitamin D
Excessive Vitamin A
Sarcoidosis

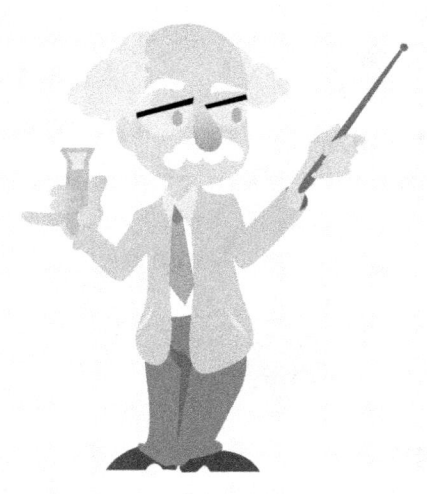

Hyperthyroidism symptoms

Mnemonic: SWEATING
S Sweating
W Weight loss
E Emotional lability
A Appetite is increased
T Tremor/Tachycardia due to AF
I Intolerance to heat/Irregular menstruation/Irritability N Nervousness
G Goitre and Gastrointestinal problems (loose stools/diarrhoea)

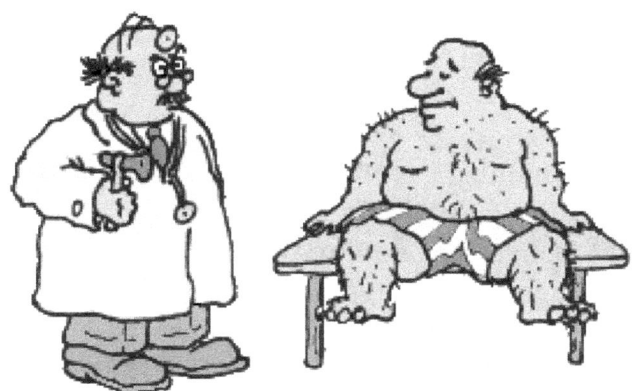

Addison's Disease: causes

Mnemonic: ADDISON

A Autoimmune (90% cases)
D Degenerative (amyloid)
D Drugs (ketoconazole)
I Infections (TB, HIV)
S Secondary (low ACTH); hypopituitarism O Others – adrenal bleeding
N Neoplasia (secondary carcinoma)

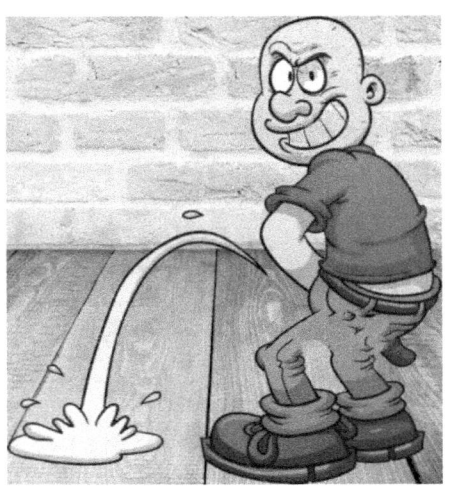

Abdomen distension Causes

Mnemonic: 6 F's
F Fat
F Fetus
F Flatus
F Faeces
F Fluid
F Flipping great tumour

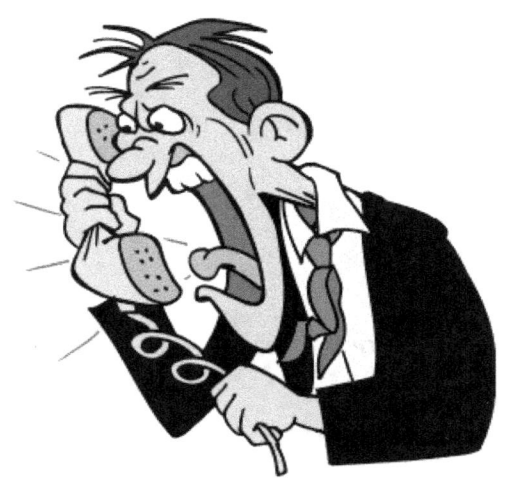

Leukaemia Symptoms and signs

LEUKEMIA

L Light skin (pallor)
E Energy decreased/Enlarged spleen, liver, lymph nodes
U Underweight
K Kidney failure
E Excess heat (fever)
M Mottled skin (haemorrhage)
I Infections
A Anaemia

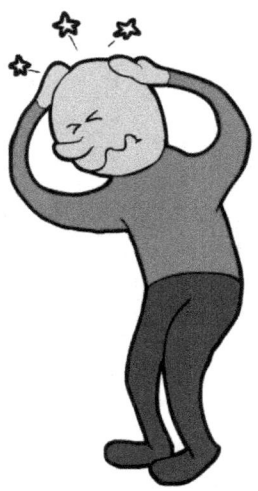

Thrombocytopenia Causes

Mnemonic: PLATELETS

P Platelet disorders: TTP, ITP, DIC L Leukaemia
A Anaemia
T Trauma
E Enlarged spleen
L Liver disease
E Ethanol
T Toxins: benzene, heparin, aspirin, chemotherapy. S Sepsis

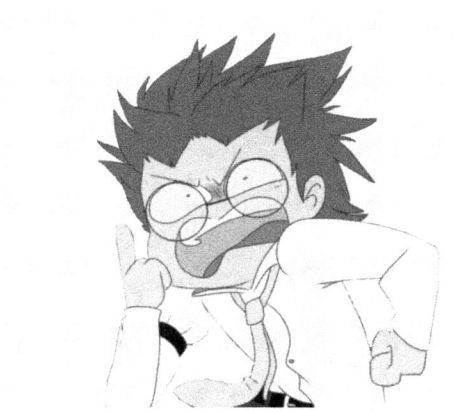

Cirrhosis severity score

ABCDE of Cirrhosis. The Child-Pugh score estimates cirrhosis severity. It is a prognosis tool.

Mnemonic: ABCDE

Albumin
Bilirubin
Coags – PT or INR
Deluge (Ascites) – Drain the Ascites
Encephalopathy

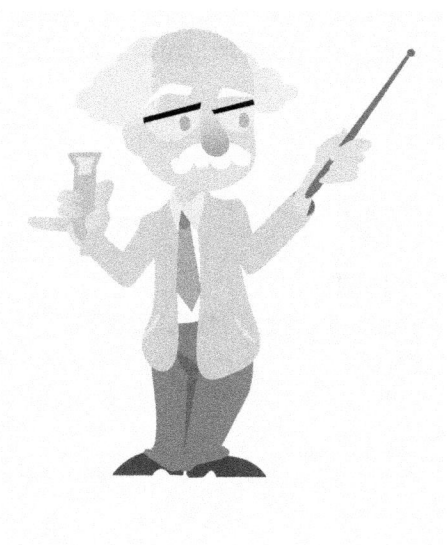

FEVER: Neuroleptic malignant syndrome

MNEMONICS : FEVER

Fever
Encephalopathy
Vital sign instability
Elevated WBC/CPK (creatine phosphokinase)
Rigidity

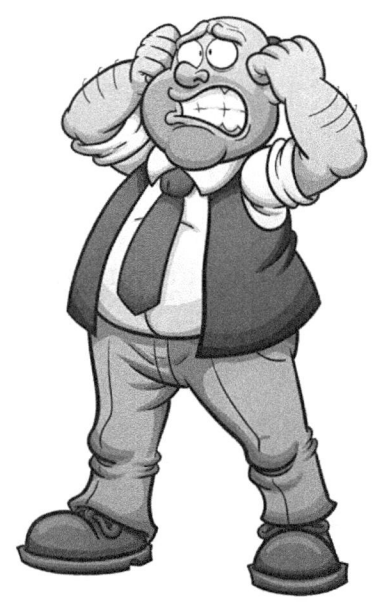

ECG Causes of ST-segment elevation: ELEVATION

MNEMONICS: ELEVATION

Electrolyte abnormalities
Left bundle branch block
Aneurysm of left ventricle
Ventricular hypertrophy
Arrhythmia disease (Brugada syndrome, ventricular tachycardia)
Takotsubo/Treatment (iatrogenic pericarditis)
Injury (myocardial infarction or cardiac contusion)
Osborne waves (hypothermia or hypocalcemia)
Non-atherosclerotic (vasospasm or Prinzmetal's angina)

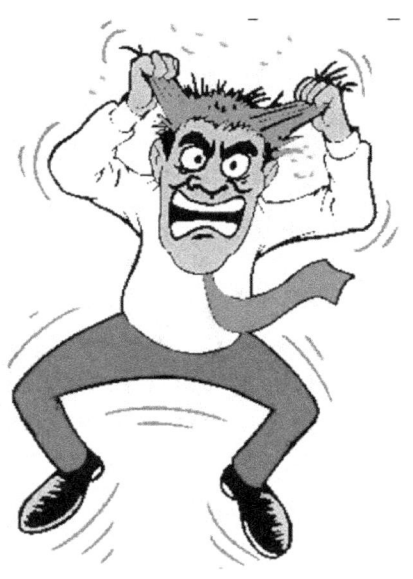

HAS-BLED Score

Mnemonic: HAS BLEED

HTN (SBP>160)
Age >65
Stroke
Bleeding history or predisposition.
Liver and Kidney dysfunction. 1pt each, a total of 2pts.
Elevated or unstable INRs, time in the therapeutic range <60%
Drugs and Alcohol. Drugs – Antiplatelets (Aspirin, Clopidogrel, NSAIDs). Alcohol – more than 8 drinks per week –1pt each, a total of 2pts.

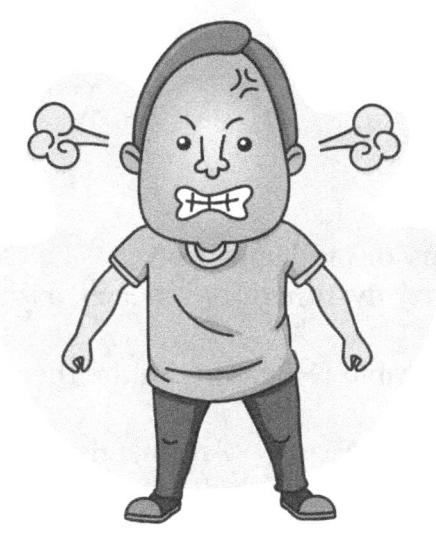

Sepsis features

mnemonics: Sepsis

Sepsis comes from Greek word meaning, to make rotten. Think septic tank.
Sepsis is an infection (suspected or confirmed) plus two of the following:
S-Sleepy, difficult to wake up, or confused: Altered Mental Status (any GCS less than 15)
E-Expiring and inspiring too much: RR>20 or PaCO2 <32 / Edema or positive fluid balance (>20 mL/kg over 24 hours)
P-Pulse >90 / pressures <90
S-Shivering (cold) or Fever: T >38.3 or <36
I-Inflammatory markers: 1) WBC >12000 or <4000 or normal WBC but >10% bands; 2) CRP > 2 SD above normal; Procalcitonin > 2 SD above normal
S-Sugars are elevated: plasma glucose >140 mg/dL or 7.7 mmol/L) in the absence of diabetes

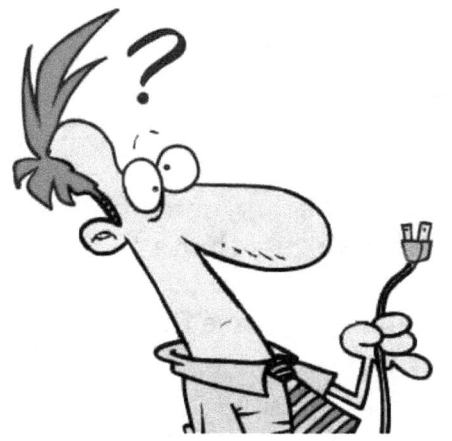

ECG: left vs. right bundle block

Mnemonic:"WiLLiaM MaRRoW":
W pattern in V1-V2 and M pattern in V3-V6 is Left bundle block.
M pattern in V1-V2 and W in V3-V6 is Right bundle block.
· Note: consider bundle branch blocks when QRS complex is wide.

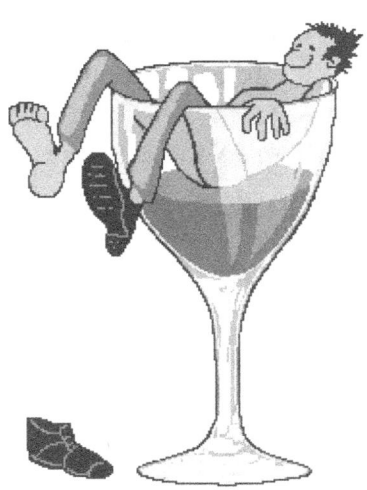

CHF: causes of exacerbation

FAILURE

Forgot medication
Arrhythmia/ Anaemia
Ischemia/ Infarction/ Infection
Lifestyle: taken too much salt
Upregulation of CO: pregnancy, hyperthyroidism
Renal failure
Embolism: pulmonary

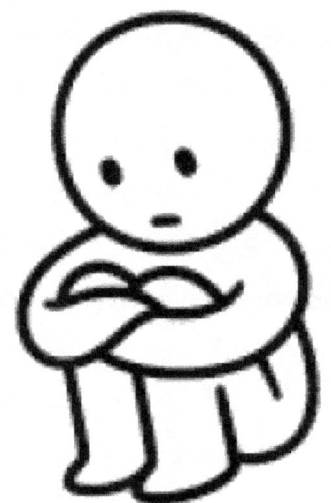

Pericarditis: EKG "PericarditiS":
PR depression in precordial leads.
ST elevation.

ECG Depressed ST-segment:

Mnemonic: DEPRESSED ST

Drooping valve (MVP)
Enlargement of LV with strain
Potassium loss (hypokalemia)
Reciprocal ST- depression (in I/W AMI)
Embolism in lungs (pulmonary embolism)
Subendocardial ischemia
Subendocardial infarct
Encephalon haemorrhage (intracranial haemorrhage)
Dilated cardiomyopathy
Shock
Toxicity of digitalis, quinidine

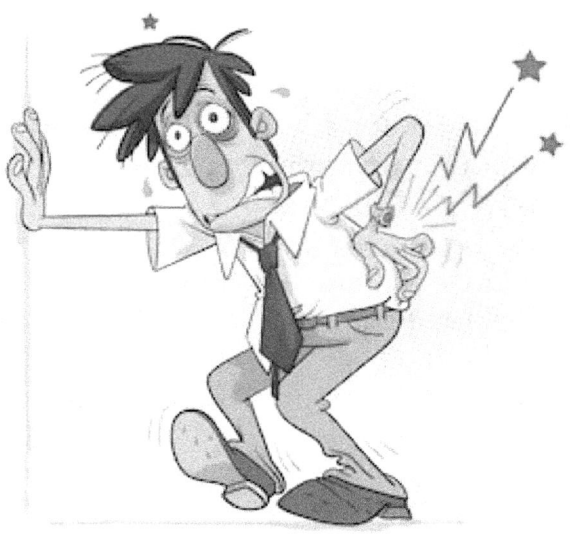

Supraventricular tachycardia Treatment

Mnemonic: ABCDE

Adenosine
Beta-blocker
Calcium channel antagonist
Digoxin
Excitation (vagal stimulation)

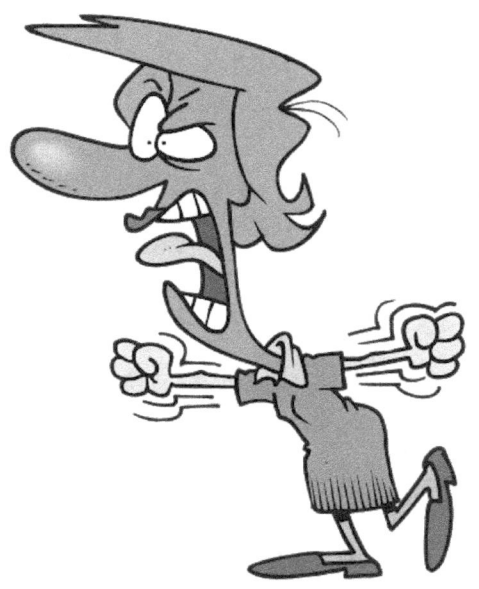

Ventricular tachycardia:

Mnemonic:LAMB

Lidocaine
Amiodarone
Mexiltene/ Magnesium
Beta-blocker

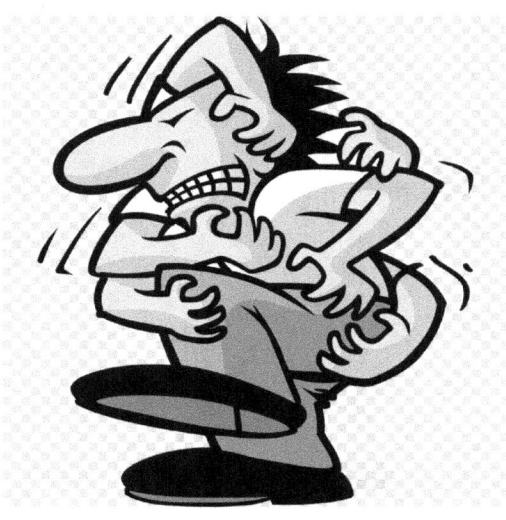

Sinus bradycardia: aetiology

Mnemonic: "SINUS BRADICARDIA"

Sleep
Infections (myocarditis)
Neap thyroid (hypothyroid)
Unconsciousness (vasovagal syncope)
Subnormal temperatures (hypothermia)
Biliary obstruction
Raised CO2 (hypercapnia)
Acidosis
Deficient blood sugar (hypoglycemia)
Imbalance of electrolytes
Cushing's reflex (raised ICP)
Aging
Rx (drugs, such as high-dose atropine)
Deep anaesthesia
Ischemic heart disease
Athletes

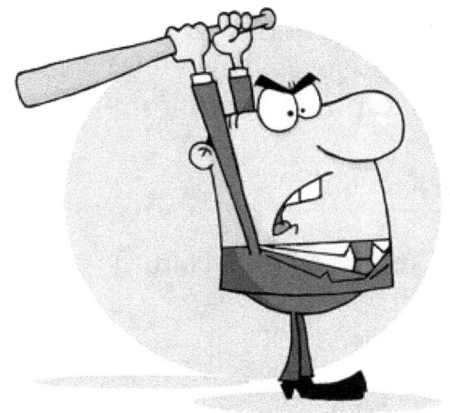

ECG: T wave inversion causes

Mnemonic:INVERT
Ischemia
Normality [esp. young, black]
Ventricular hypertrophy
Ectopic foci [eg calcified plaques]
RBBB, LBBB
Treatments [digoxin]

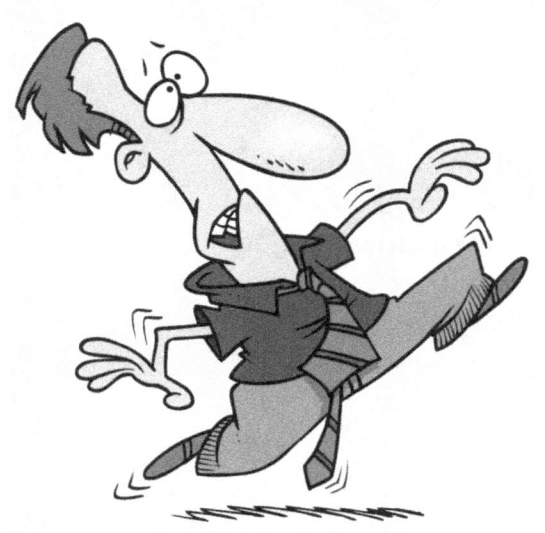

Myocardial infarctions:

Mnemonic:INFARCTIONS

IV access
Narcotic analgesics (eg morphine, pethidine)
Facilities for defibrillation (DF)
Aspirin/ Anticoagulant (heparin)
Rest
Converting enzyme inhibitor
Thrombolysis
IV beta blocker
Oxygen 60%
Nitrates
Stool Softeners

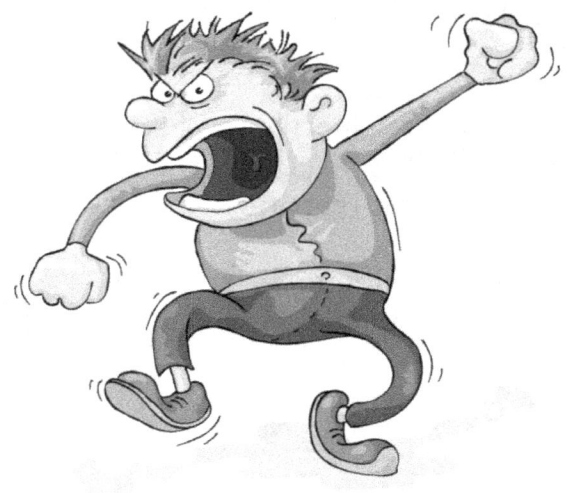

Atrial fibrillation: management

Mnemonic :ABCD
Anti-coagulate
Beta-block to control rate
Cardiovert
Digoxin

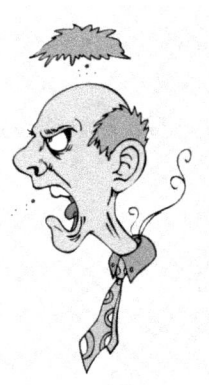

Differential diagnosis checklist

Mnemonic:"I VINDICATE":

Iatrogenic
Vascular
Infectious
Neoplastic
Degenerative/ Drugs
Inflammatory/ Idiopathic
Congenital
Allergic/ Autoimmune
Traumatic
Endocrinal & metabolic

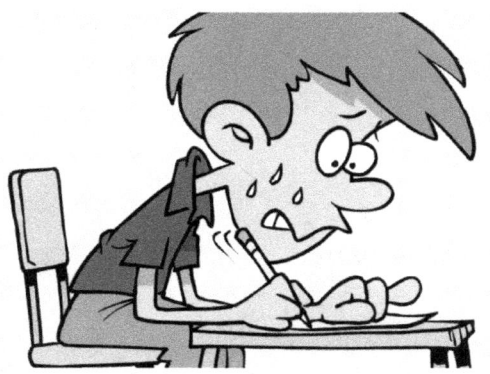

Coma: conditions to exclude as cause

Mnemonic: MIDAS
Meningitis
Intoxication
Diabetes
Air (respiratory failure)
Subdural/ Subarachnoid hemorrhage

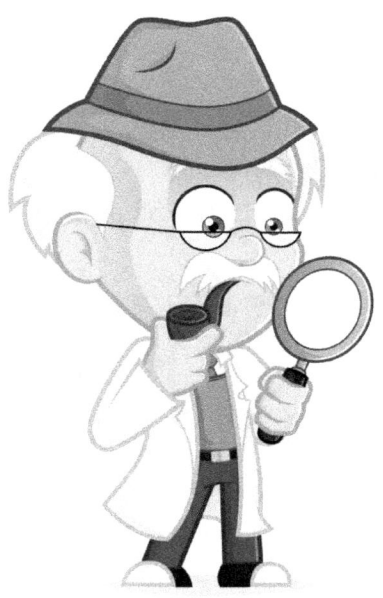

Asthma: management of acute severe

Mnemonic:"O S#!T":
Oxygen (high dose: >60%)
Salbutamol (5mg via oxygen-driven nebuliser)
Hydrocortisone (or prednisolone)
Ipratropium bromide (if life threatening)
Theophylline (or preferably aminophylline-if life threatening)

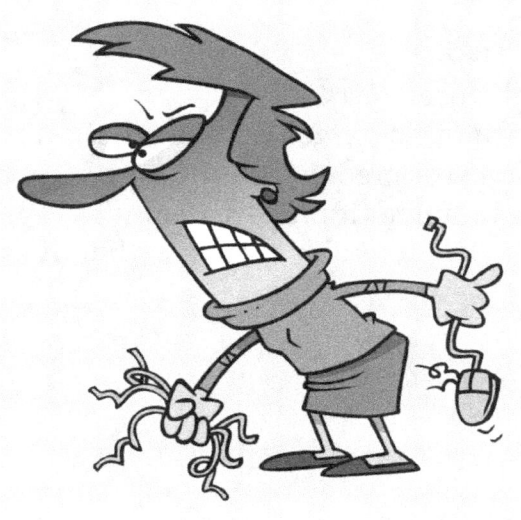

RLQ pain: differential

Mnemonic: APPENDICITIS

Appendicitis/ Abscess PID/ Period Pancreatitis Ectopic/ Endometriosis Neoplasia Diverticulitis Intussusception Crohns Disease/ Cyst (ovarian) IBD Torsion (ovary) Irritable Bowel Syndrome Stones

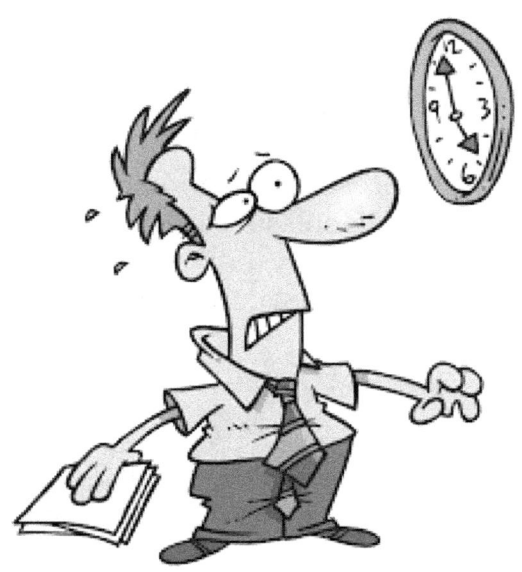

Ulcerative colitis: definition of a severe attack

A STATE

Anemia less than 10g/dl
Stool frequency greater than 6 stools/day with blood
Temperature greater than 37.5
Albumin less than 30g/L
Tachycardia greater than 90bpm
ESR greater than 30mm/hr

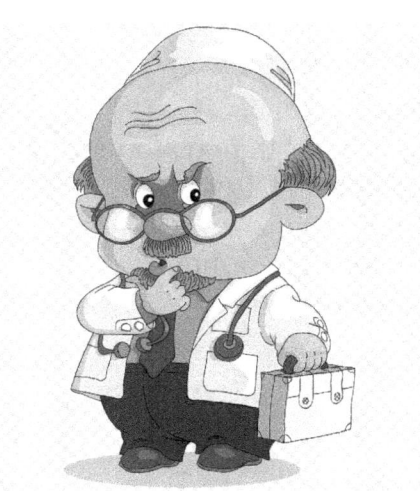

Bilirubin: common causes for increased levels

Mnemonic:"HOT Liver":
Hemolysis
Obstruction
Tumor
Liver disease

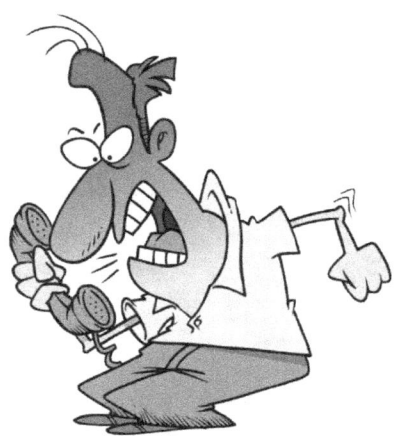

Dysphagia: differential

Mnemonic:DISPHAGIA

Disease of mouth and tonsils/ Diffuse oesophageal spasm/ Diabetes mellitus
Intrinsic lesion
Scleroderma
Pharyngeal disorders/ Palsy-bulbar-MND
Achalasia
Heart: eft atrium enlargement
Goitre/ myesthenia Gravis/ mediastinal Glands
Infections
American trypanosomiasis (chagas disease)

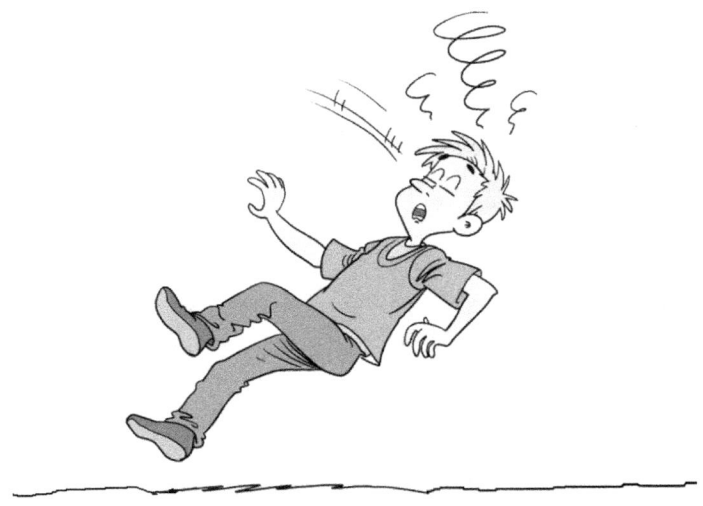

Dry mouth: differential

Mnemonic:"DRI":

Drugs/ Dehydration
Renal failure/ Radiotherapy
Immunological (Sjogren's)/ Intense emotions

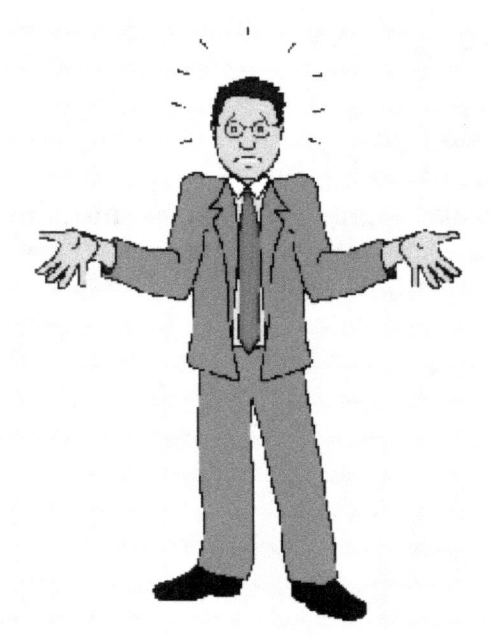

Hepatic encephalopathy: precipitating factors

Mnemonic: HEPATICS
Hemorrhage in GIT/ Hyperkalemia
Excess protein in diet
Paracentesis
Acidosis/ Anemia
Trauma
Infection
Colon surgery
Sedatives

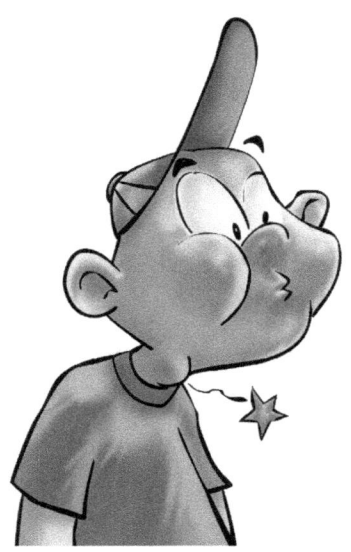

Splenomegaly: causes

Mnemonic :CHIMP

Cysts
Haematological (eg CML, myelofibrosis)
Infective (eg viral (IM), bacterial)
Metabolic/ Misc (eg amyloid, Gauchers)
Portal hypertension

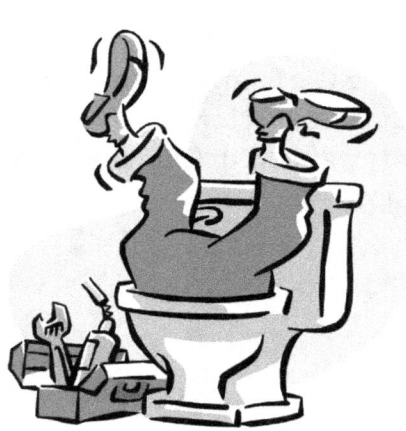

Clubbing: causes

Mnemonic:Clubbing

C : cardiac (R -> L shunt)
L : lung (tumor, fibrosis)
U : ulcerative colitis (also Crohn's disease less commonly)
B : bronchiectasis
B : benign mesothelioma
I : inherited; idiopathic; IBD
N : neurogenic tumors
G : GI (cirrhosis, crohn's, UC)

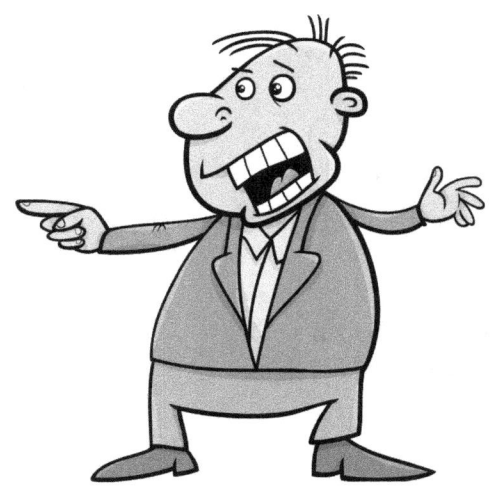

Increased anion gap acidosis

Mnemonic : MUDPIES

M : methanol
U : uremia
D : diabetes
P : paraldehyde
I : idiopathic (lactic acidosis)
E : ethylene glycol
S : salicylates

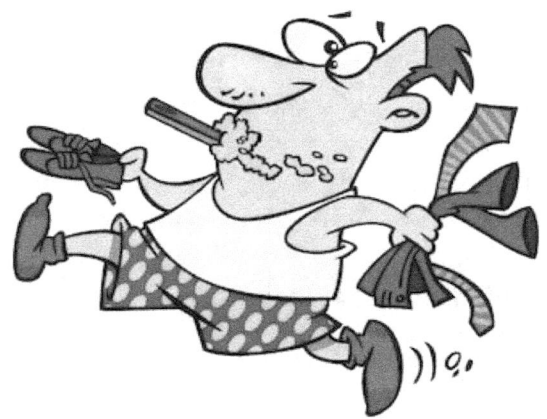

Normal anion gap acidosis

Mnemonic : USED CAR

U : uterosigmoidostomy
S : saline administration (in the face of renal dysfunction)
E : endocrine (Addisons, spironolactone, triamterene, amiloride,
primary hyperparathyroidism)
D : diarrhea

C : carbonic anhydrase inhibitors
A : ammonium chloride
R : renal tubular acidosis

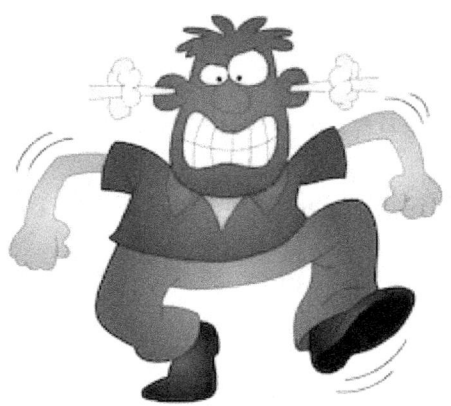

Proven MI.. should be met by M.O.N.A.

Mnemonic: MONA

M = morphine
O = oxygen
N = nitrates
A = aspirin

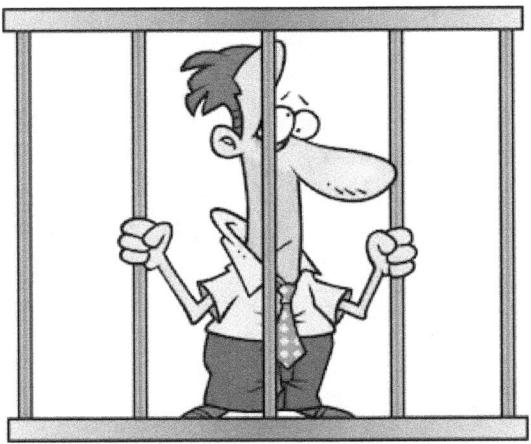

Symptoms of hyperthyroidism

Mnemonic: SWEATING

S: Sweating

T: Tremor or Tachycardia

I: Intolerance to heat, Irregular menstruation, and Irritability

N: Nervousness

G: Goiter and Gastrointestinal (loose stools/diarrhea).

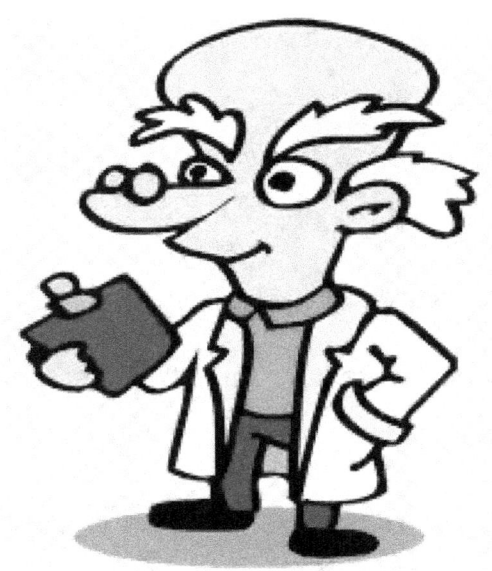

Jaundice causes

Medical causes

Medical Doctors Aren't Very Happy

Malignancy – lymphoma, hepatocellular carcinoma
Drugs – oral contraceptive pill, IVDA, overdose
Alcohol – liver disease, cirrhosis, acute alcoholic hepatitis
Viruses – hepatitis A, B, C, EBV, CMV
Haematological – haemolytic anaemia
Surgical causes

Surgeons ARe Not Much better

Stones – painful jaundice
Antibiotics/Anaesthetic effect
Reabsorption of haematoma
Nodal obstruction – painful or painless
Malignancy of pancreatic head

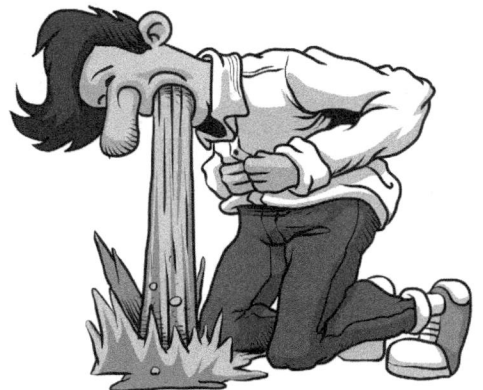

Esophageal cancer: risk factors

Mnemonic:ABCDEF

Achalasia

Barret's esophagus

Corrosive esophagitis

Diverticuliis

Esophageal web

Familial

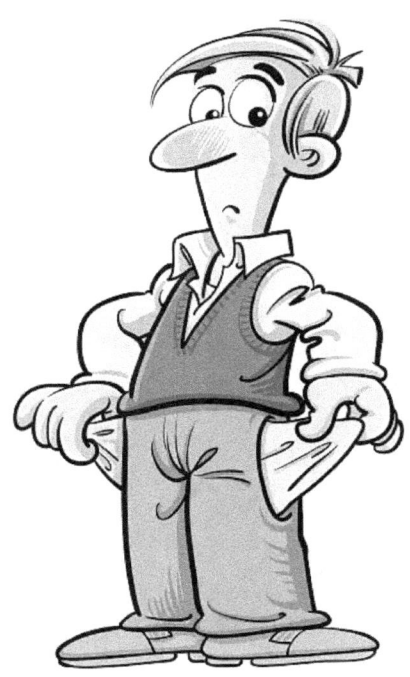

Head Trauma: rapid neuro

Mnemonic: 12 P's

Psychological (mental) status

Pupils: size, symmetry, reaction

Paired ocular movements

Papilloedema

Pressure (BP, increased ICP)

Pulse and rate

Paralysis, Paresis

Pyramidal signs

Pin prick sensory response

Pee (incontinent)

Patellar reflex

Ptosis

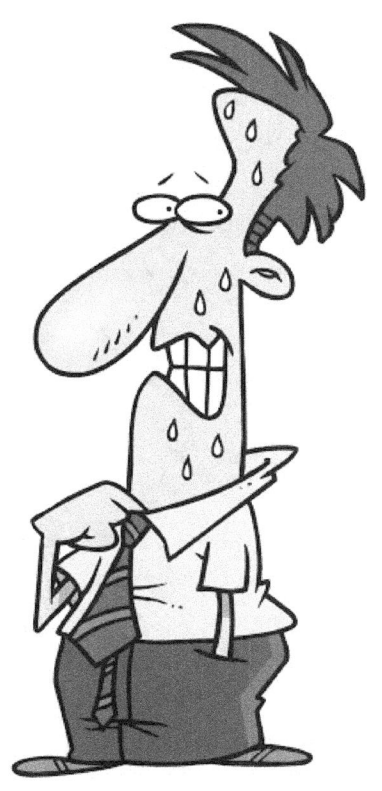

Horner Syndrome

Mnemonic: Horny PAMELA

Ptosis

Anhydrosis

Miosis

Enophthalmos

Loss of ciliary-spinal reflex

Anisocoria

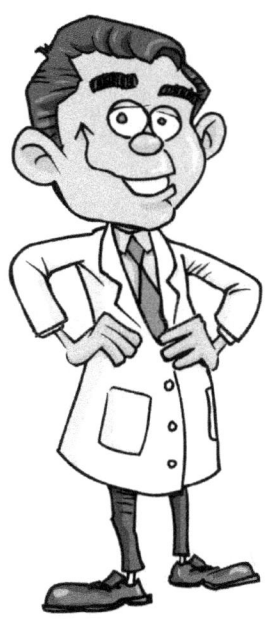

Pulmonary Edema: Treatment

Mnemonic: LMNOP

Lasix

Morphine

Nitro

Oxygen

Position/Positive pressure ventilation

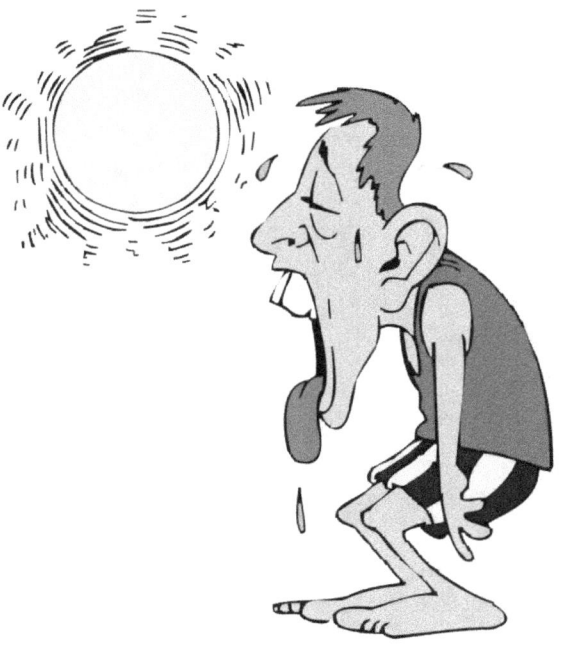

DKA

Triad of DKA is D.K.A.
Diabetics with sugar more than 14 mmol/l
Ketonemia +ve at 1:2 dilution or Ketonuria at least 3+
Acidosis with pH less than 7.3 or HCO3- less than 15 mmol
Note: Remember: 14 and 15
1.2. The signs and symptoms of DKA is D.K.A.
D = Delirium, diuresis, dehydrated (3D)
K = Kussmaul breathing, ketotic breath (2K)
A = Abdominal pain (1A)
1.3. The precipitating factors of DKA is SSSSS..................
S = Sepsis
S = Surgery
S = Stress
S = Sugar high due to skipped insulin
S = Substance abuse, dope, alcohol

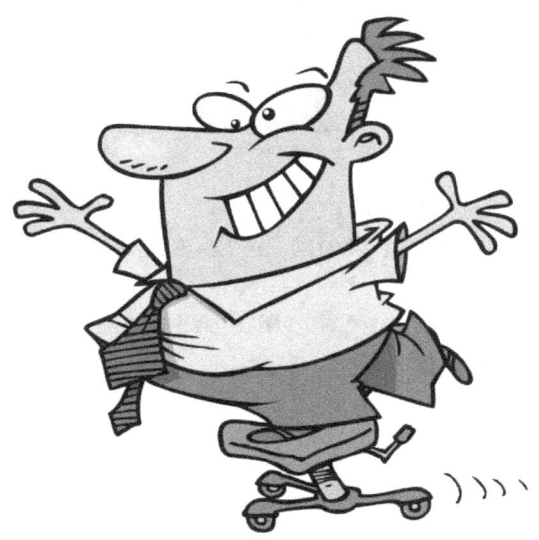

Interventions for critically ill patients in ED.

FAST HUG
The mnemonic stands for:

F = Fluid Resuscitation and balance
A = Analgesia
S = Sedation
T = Thromboembolic prophylaxis

H = Head-of-bed elevation
U = stress Ulcer prophylaxis, and
G = Glucose/glycemic control.

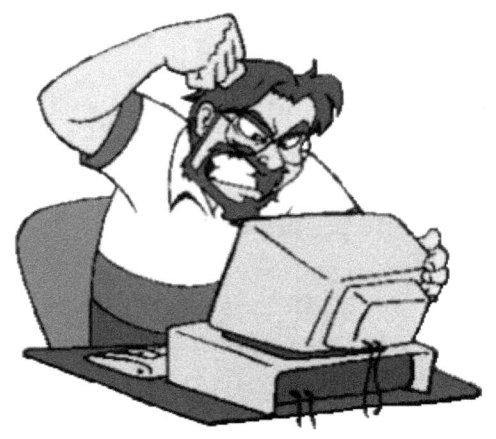

San Francisco Syncope Rule

Mnemonic:CHESS

C = history of Congestive heart failure,
H = Hematocrit <30%,
E =" Electrocardiogram abnormality,
S = Shortness of breath, or
S = Systolic blood pressure <90 mm Hg (the criteria can be remembered by the mnemonic, CHESS).

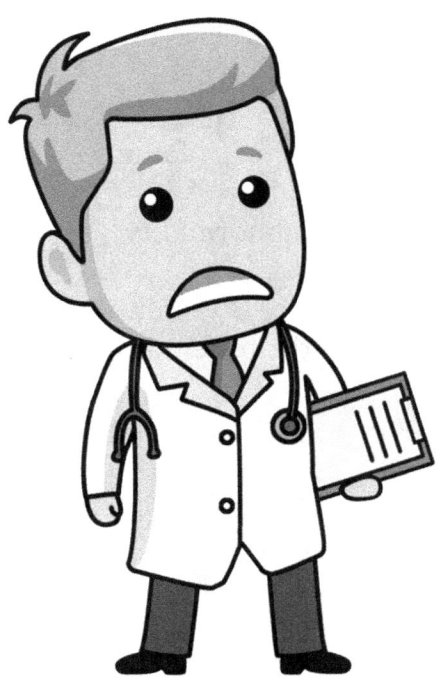

Massage Splenomegaly causes

Mnemonic: 3 M

= Malaria
= Myeloid leukemia (chronic)
= Myelofibrosis

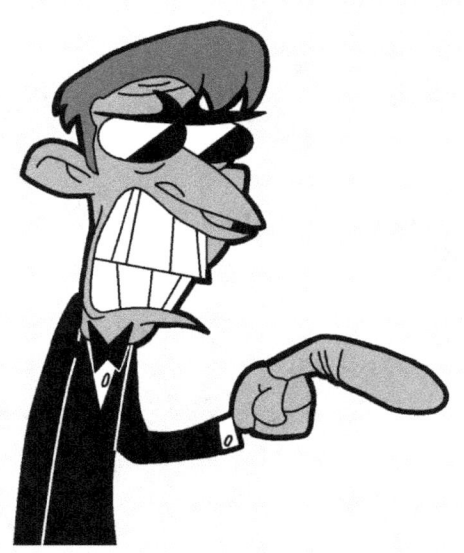

Causes of raised hemidiaphragm on CXR

Mnemonic 5 P

P = Pulled - "Pulled" Upwards Active due to lung fibrosis pulling up the diaphragm passively or lung diseases causing volume loss for example, atelectasis of lower lobes and pneumonectomy
P = Pushed - Pushed upwards due to hepatomegaly, abscess, ascites, pancreatitis, pregnancy
P = Perforate - "Perforation" due to diaphragmatic rupture with herniation of bowels into thorax
P = Phrenic nerve paralysis
P = Pseudo - "pseudodiaphragm" subpulmonic Effusion

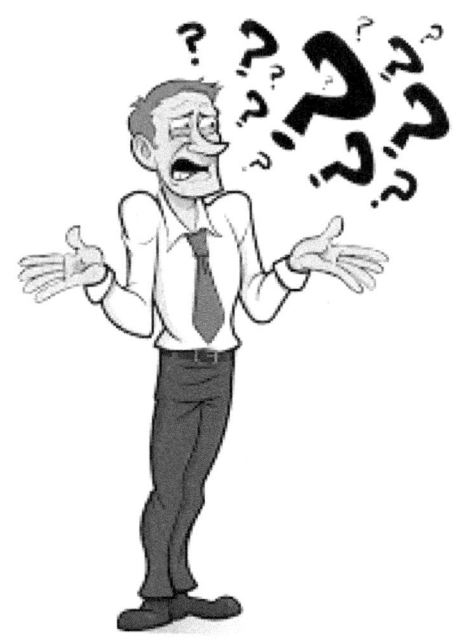

JVP: raised JVP differential

Mnemonic: PQRST(EKG waves)

Pericardial effusion
Quantity of fluid raised (fluid over load)
Right heart failure
Superior vena caval obstruction
Tricuspid stenosis/Tricuspid regurgitation/Tamponade (cardiac)

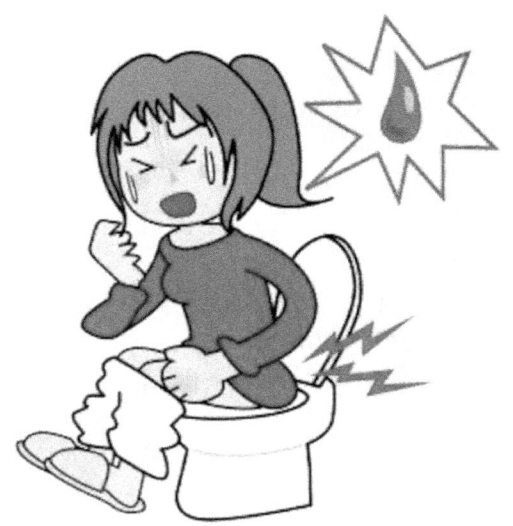

DDx of Lower GI Bleeding:

Mnemonic: High DRAIN

Hemorrhoids
Diverticulosis / Diverticulits
Radiation colitis
AVM
Infection / IBD / Ischemic gut
Neoplasm

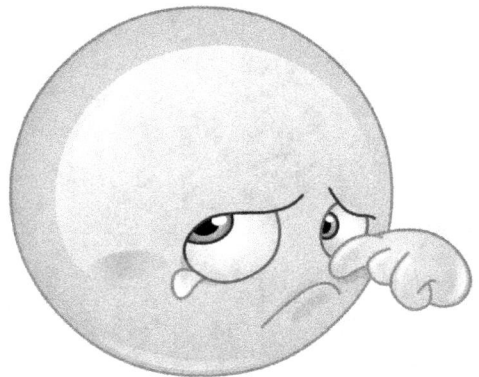

DDx of Bowel Obstruction

Mnemonic :HANG IV
H ernia
A dhesions
N eoplasm
G allstone ileus
I ntussusception
V olvulus

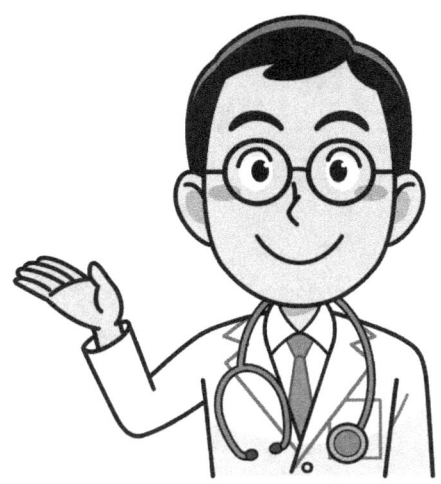

Bowel obstruction symptoms

Mnemonic: AVOID

AVOID = Bowel obstruction symptoms
A bdominal pain
V omiting
O bstipation, i.e. not passing gas
I ncreased bowel sounds
D istention of the abdomen

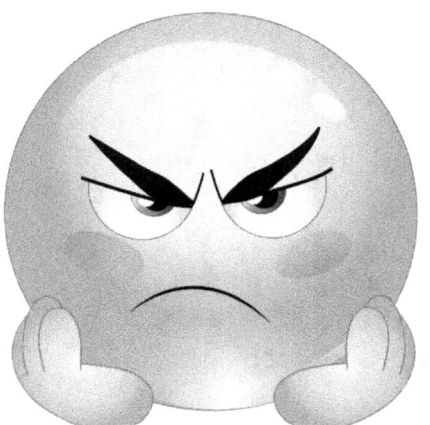

Mnemonic for Differential Diagnosis of Hyperkalemia:

Mnemonic: ART x 3

Artifact, e.g. hemolytic sample
ACEi treatment
Addison's

Renal failure
Rhabdomyolysis
RTA type 1 (distal RTA)

Tumor lysis syndrome
Transcellular shift, e.g. in acidosis
Treatment – urgent treatment required if K+ higher than 6

Boo

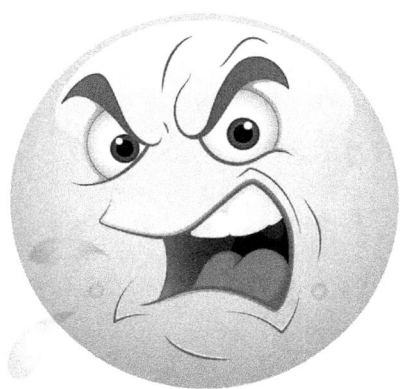

Proximal myopathy: causes

Mnemonic: OCD

. Osteomalacia
. Dermatomyositis/Drugs
. Cushing disease/carcinoma

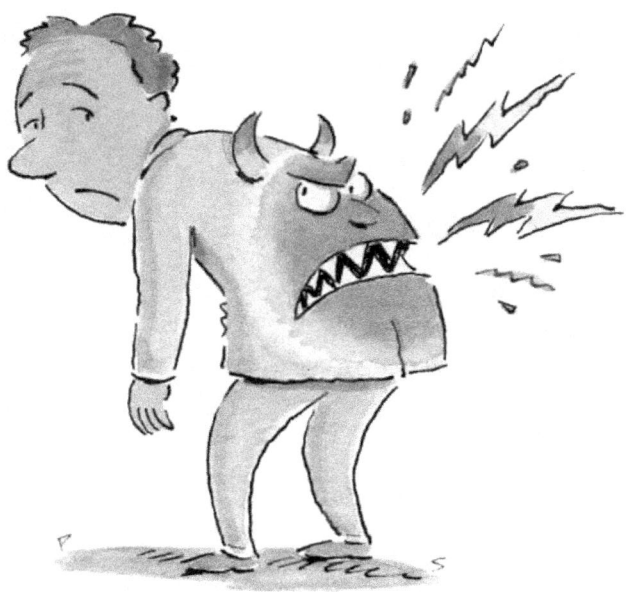

Secondary nephrotic syndrome:Causes

Mnemonic : DAVID
Diabetes mellitus
Amyloidosis
Vasculitis
Infections
Drugs

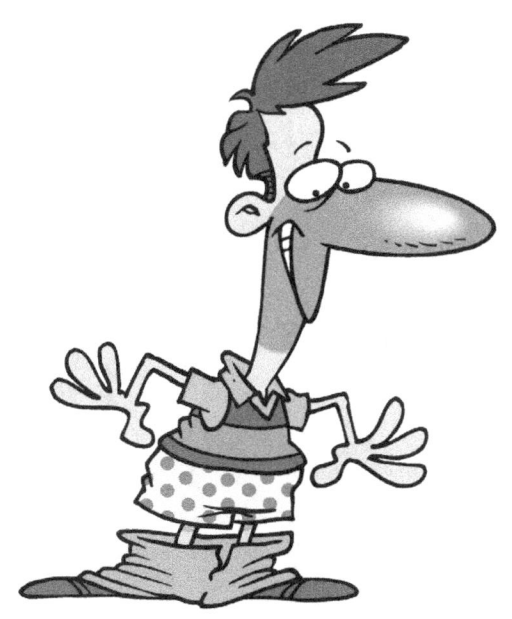

Papilloedema; causes

Mnemonic: BATS

.Being Intracranial hypertension/Bleed
. Abscess
. Tumour
. Space-occupying lesion

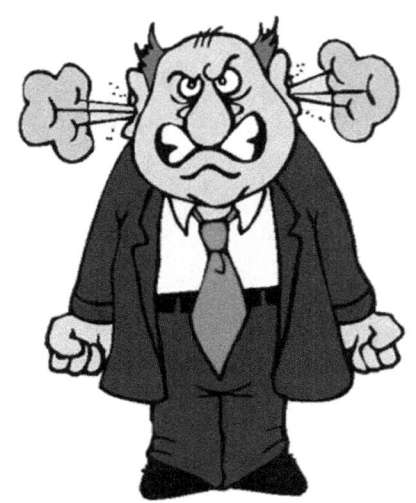

Ptosis: causes

Mnemonic: The Hypotonic Muscle Can't Move

. Third nerve palsy
. Horner syndrome
. Myasthenia gravis
. Congenital
. Myotonic dystrophy

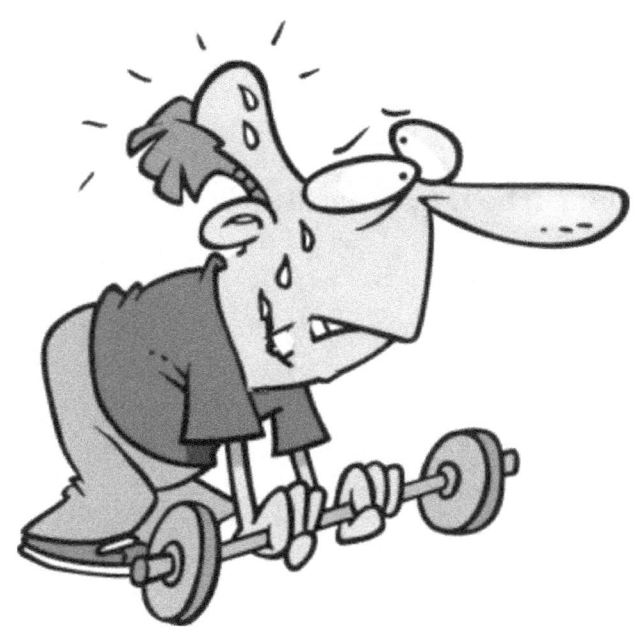

Macrocyclic anemia causes

Mnemonic:ABCDEF

Alcohol (liver diseases)
B12 deficiency
Compensatory reticulocytosis (blood loss and hemolysis)
Drug (cytotoxic drugs and AZT)/ Dysplasia (marrow disorders)
Endocrine (hypothyroidism)
Folate deficieny/ Fetus (pregnancy)

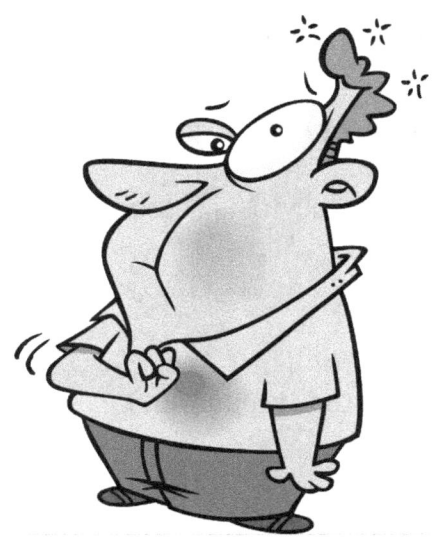

Splenomegaly causes

" CHINA "

Congestion – portal hypertension
Haematological – haemolytic anaemia, sickle cell disease
Infection – Malaria, EBV, CMV, HIV
Neoplasm – CML, myelofibrosis, lymphoma
Autoimmune – RA, sarcoidosis, amyloidosis

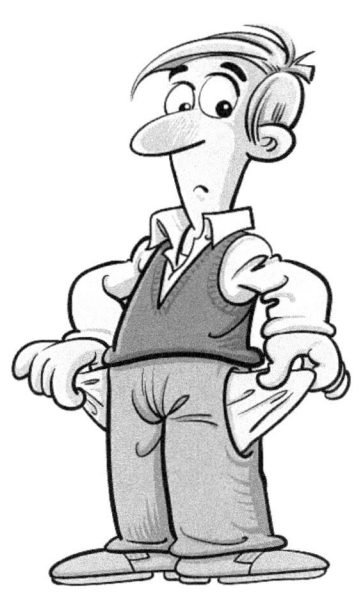

Nephrotic syndrome : Features

Mnemonic: NEPHROTIC

Na+ & water retention
Edema
Proteinuria > 3.5g/day
Hyperlipidemia
Renal vein thrOmbosis
Thrombotic and thromboembolic complications
Infection with staph. N pneumococci
Coagulable state

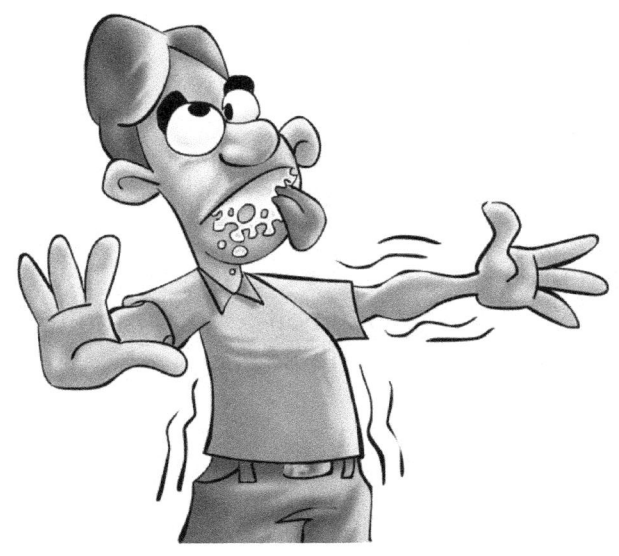

Pyrexia Unknown Origin ;

Mnemonic : IMAGINE

Infections:
 Malignancy
Automimmune Diseases
Granulomas (Sarcoidosis, Crohn's disease)
Iatrogenic (Drug fever, Thrombophlebitis)
Nurses, Doctors and all paramedical staff: factitious fever

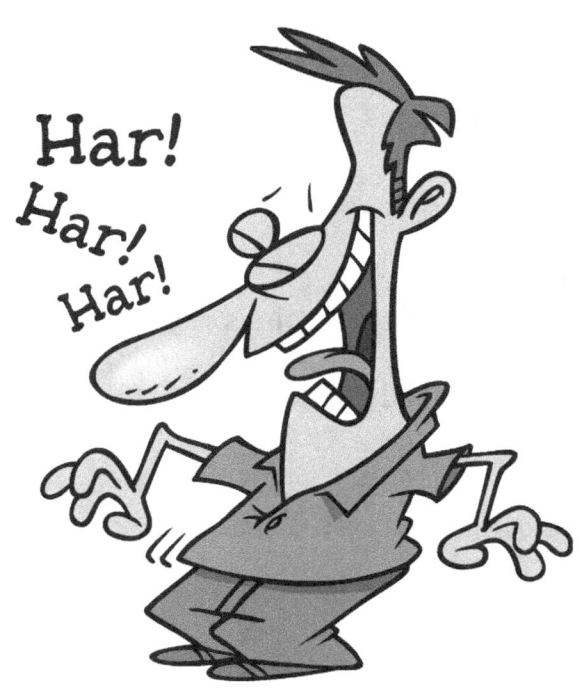

Pheochromocytoma : Clinical features

Mnemonic: 5P's

1. Pounding headache
2. Palpitations
3. Perspiration
4. Paroxysmal hypertension (usually)
5. Pain (abdominal pain)

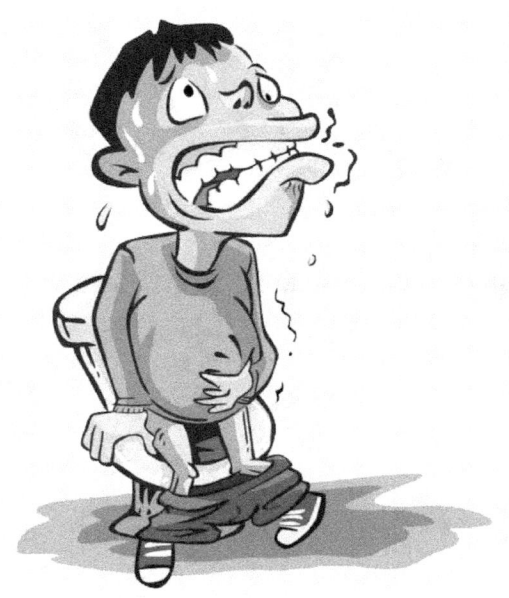

GBS

Mnemonic: 4 A's
Acute inflammatory demyelinating polyneuropathy
Ascending paralysis
Autonomic neuropathy
Arrythmias

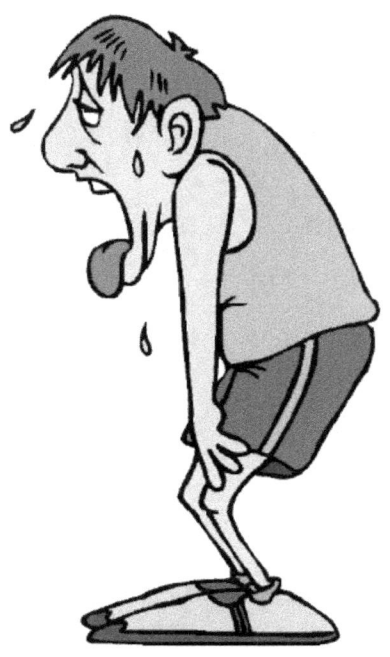

DELIRIUM

Mnemonic: DELERIUM

Degenerative
Epilepsy (post ictal states)
Liver failure
Intracranial injury
Rheumatic chorea
Infections- Pneumonia, Septicemia
Uremia
Metabolic- Electrolyte imbalance

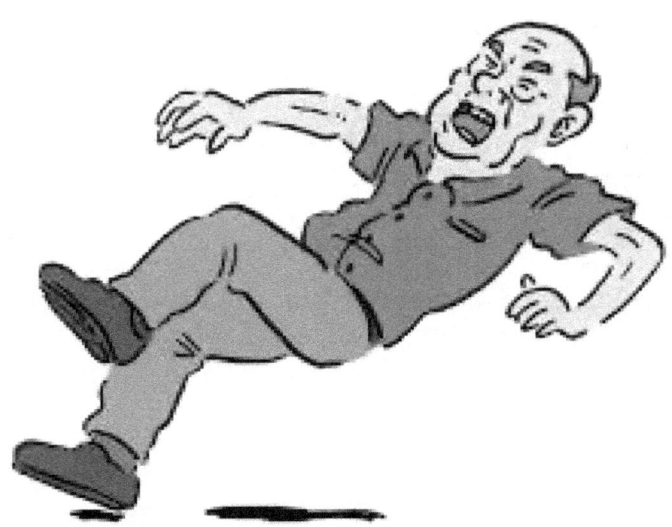

Hypokalemia

Mnemonic:BAD LOAD

Barters/Conns syndrome(hyperaldosteronism)
Alkalosis
Diuretics
Laxative abuse
Other causes: insulin overdose
Acute glucose load
Diarrhoea

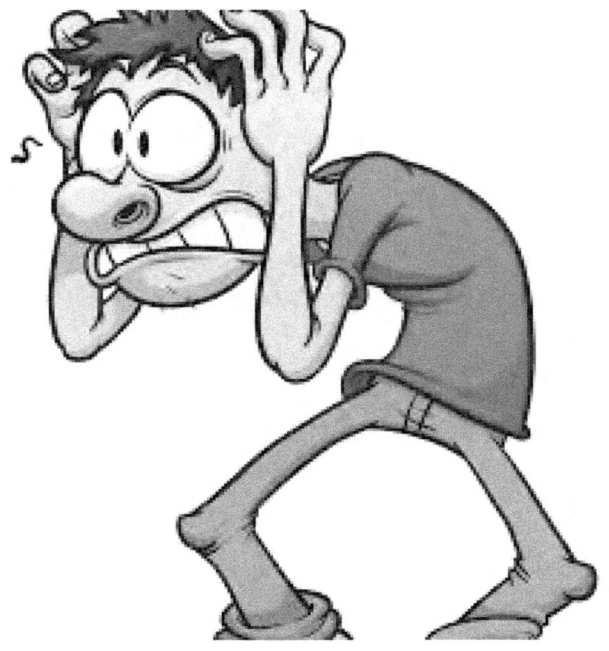

Morphine: side-effects

Mnemonic: MORPHINE

M:- Myosis,
O:- Out of it (sedation),
R:- Respiratory depression,
P:- Pneumonia (aspiration),
H:- Hypotension,
I:- Infrequency (constipation, urinary retention),
N:- Nausea,
E:- Emesis

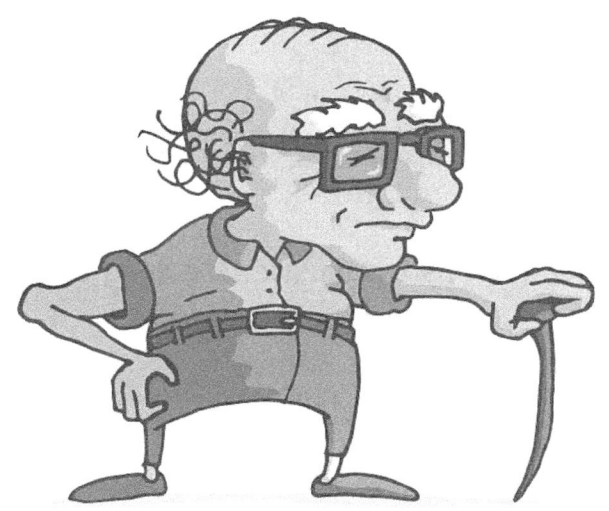

Hepatomegaly

Mnemonic: 3 CCC

. Cancer (metastatic)
. Cirrhosis
. Congestive cardiac failure

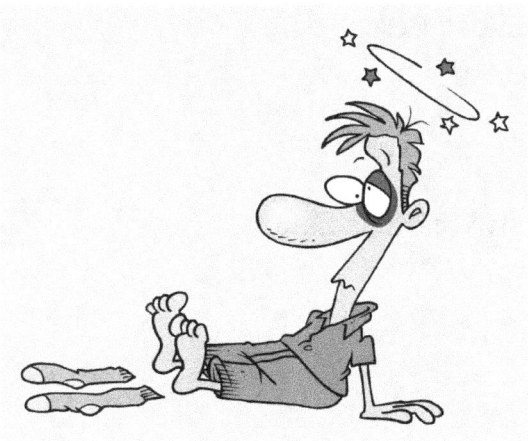

Bradycardia

Mnemonic: Bradycardia Means A Slow Heart

. Beta Blockers
. Myocardial infarction
. Active individuals
. Sinoatrial disease
. Hypothyroidism

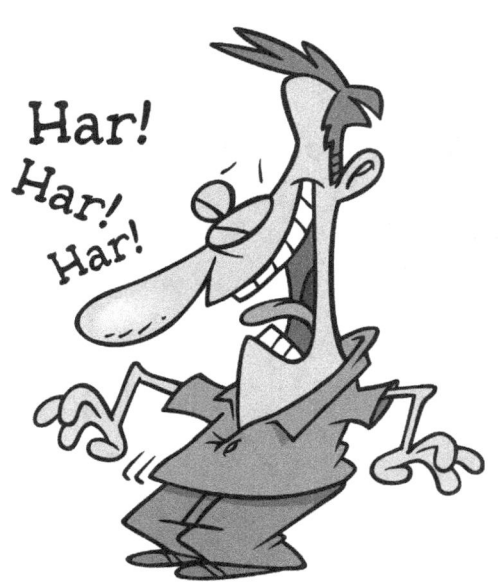

Ectopics

Mnemonic: Irregular Hearts Are Dangerous

Ischaemic/idiopathic
Hyperthyroid
Atrial enlargement
Digoxin

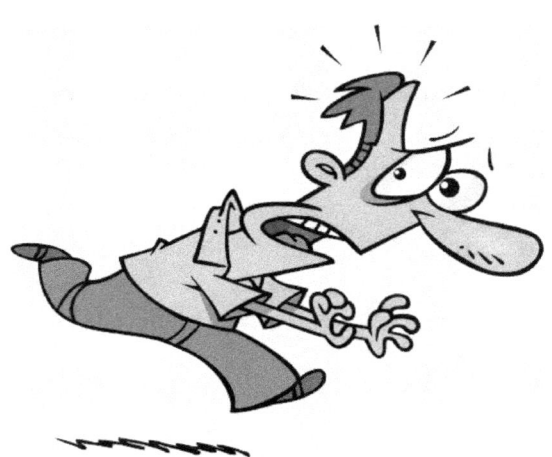

Cerebellar dysfunction causes

Mnemonic: My Balance Problem Affects Function

. Multiple sclerosis
. Brain stem vascular lesions
. Posterior fossa space occupying lesions/paraneoplastic syndrome
. Alcohol cerebellar degeneration.

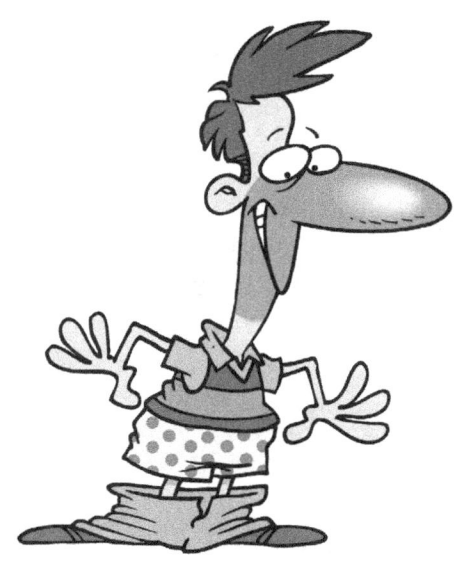

Raised JVP

Mnemonic: Fluid Retention causes high venous pressure

Fluid retention
Regurgitation (tricuspid)
Cor pulmonale
Heart block
Vena cava obstruction
Pericardial effusion/pericarditis (constrictive)

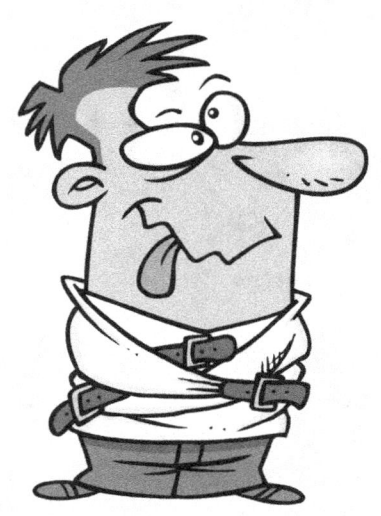

Collapse on a psychiatric ward

Mnemonic: FLAT

Fits
Long QT
Acute Intermittent porphyria
Tricyclics antidepressants overdose

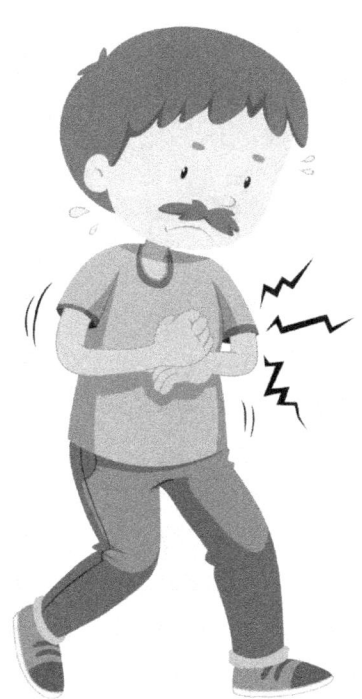

Impaired consciousness in alcohol abusers

Mnemonic: Boozers Fall Into The Empty Gutter

Brain bleed (subdural)
Fits (withdrawal/epileptic)
Infections (meningitis)
Trauma
Encephalopathy (Wernicke/hepatic)
Gastrointestinal bleeding

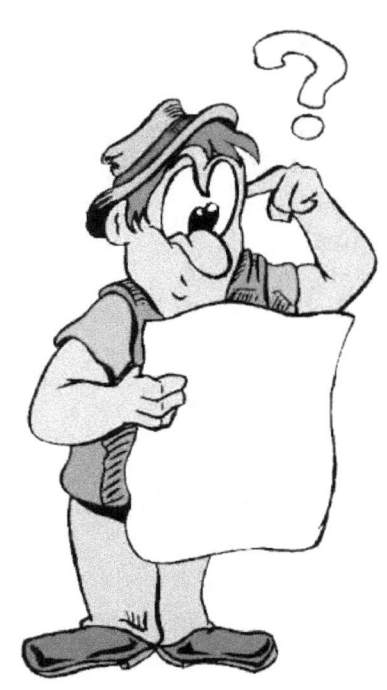

Papilloedema

Mnemonic: STAB

Space-occupying lesion
Tumour
Abscess
Bleed/benign intracranial hypertension

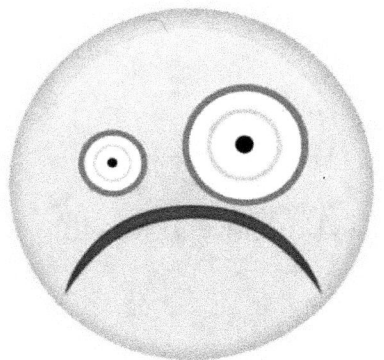

Paraplegia

Mnemonic:ABC

Atlantiaxial subluxation
Bleed (into the cord)
Cord compression/truma

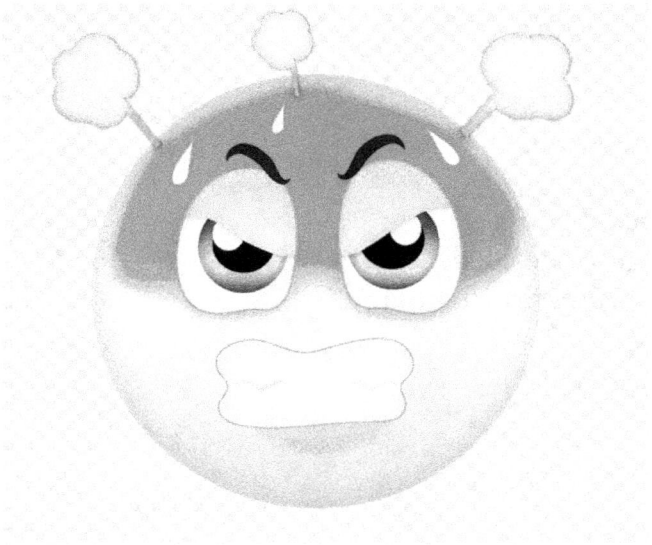

Sensory ataxia

Mnemonic: Sensation Shit & Totally Crap

Subacute combined degeneration
Spinocebellar disease
Tabes dorslis
Cervical myelopathy

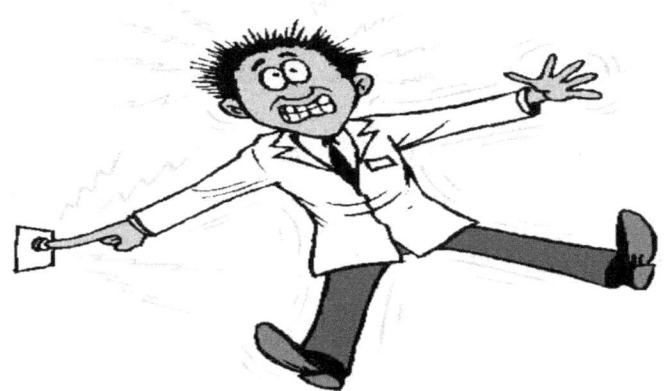

Sixth nerve palsy

Mnemonic: MMR Not My Vaccine

Mononeuritis multiplex
Multiple sclerosis
Raised ICP
Neoplasm
Myasthenia gravis
Vascular

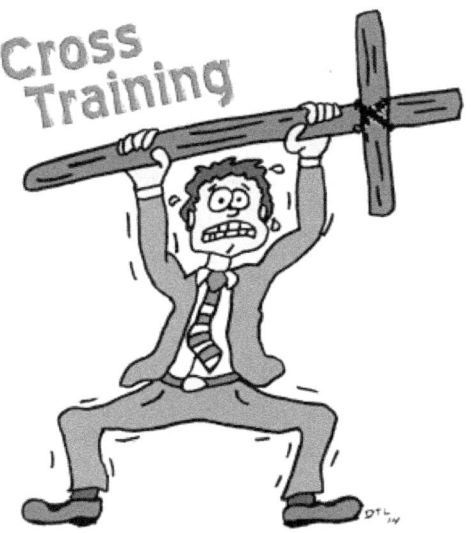

Spastic Paraparesis

Mnemonic: Major Cord Trauma Buggers Mobility

. Multiple sclerosis
. Cord compression
. Trauma
. Birth injury
. MND

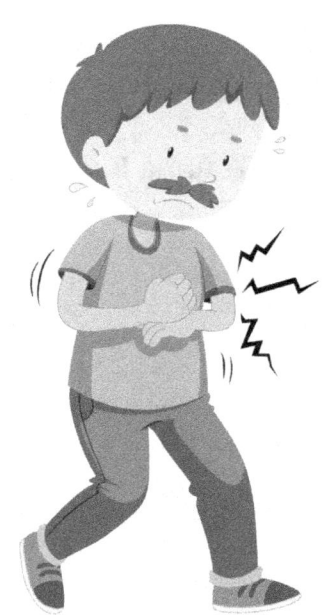

Third nerve palsy

Mnemonic: Partial & Minimal Visual Movement

. Posterior communicating artery aneurysm
. Mono neuritis multiplex
. Vascular lesions
. Multiple scelorosis
. Myasthenia gravis

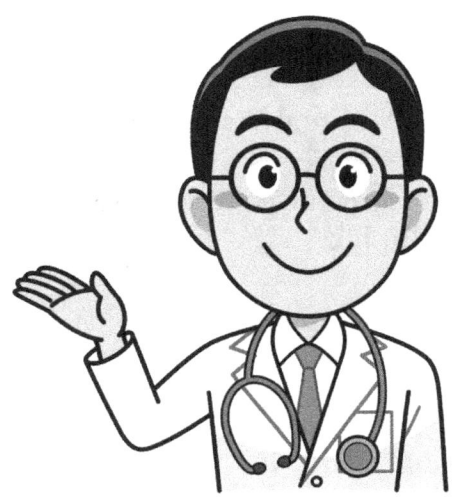

Ascites

Mnemonic: 5 Cs

. Cirrhosis
. Cancer
. Cardiac failure
. Caval compression
. Constrictive pericarditis

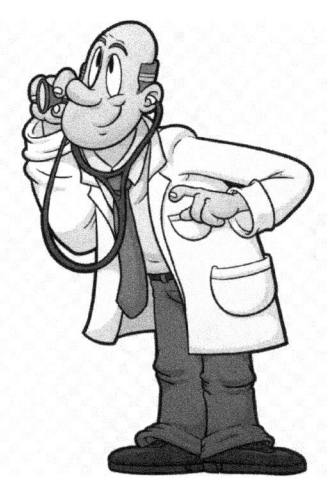

Cholestatic jaundice

Mnemonic: Drugs Can Precipitate Hepatic Obstruction

. Drugs
. Cirrhosis
. Pregnancy
. Hepatitis
. Obstruction

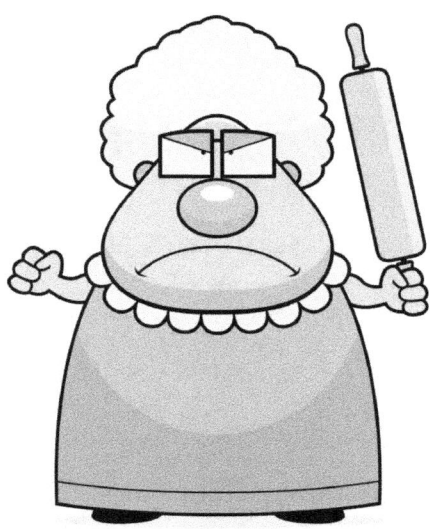

Chronic Liver Disease

Mnemonic: Cirrhosis Has Always Been Corelated With Alcohol

. Chronic active hepatitis
. Haemochromatosis/Hepatitis
. Alpha 1 antritrypsin deficiency
. Budd-chiari syndrome/biliary cirrhosis
. Wilson Disease
. Alcohol

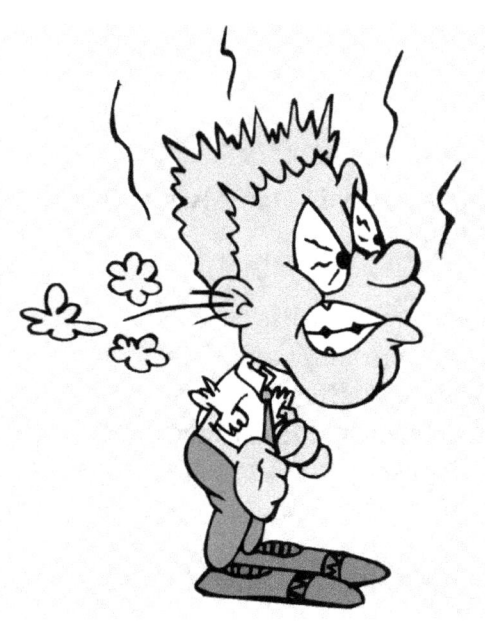

Diverticular disease : clinical features

Mnemonic:Bald Poo

. Bleeding (rectal)
. Altered biwel Disease
. Left iliac fossa
. Diarrhea
. Perforation
. Obstruction
. Other (fistula)

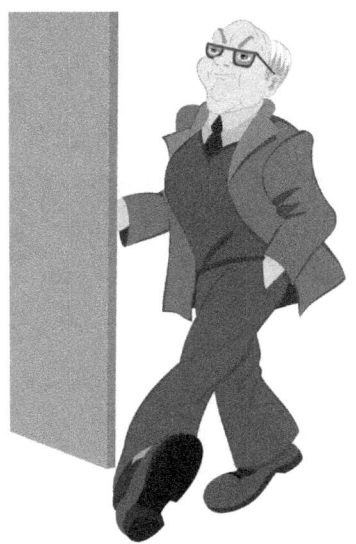

Upper Gastrointestinal bleeding

Mnemonic:Upper Gastrointestinal oesophageal varices & tear

.Ulcers (gastric)
. Gastritis
. Oesophageal
. Varices
. Tear (Mallory-Weiss tear)

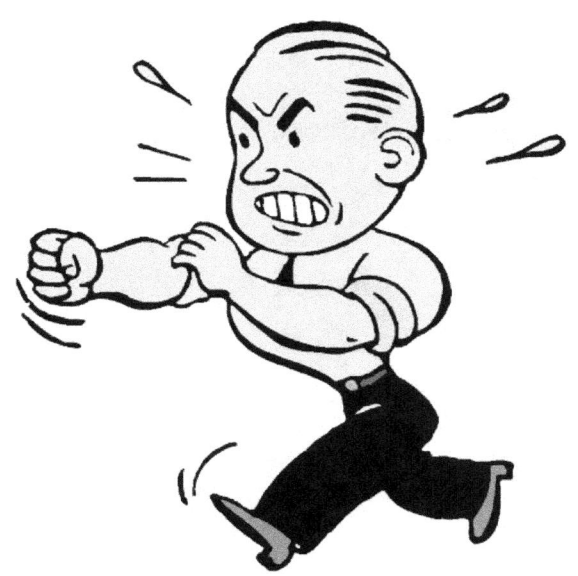

Hepatic encephalopathy : precipitants

Mnemonic: Bad infection can damage hepatic

- Bleed
- Azotemia
- Drugs
- Infections
- Constipation
- Dehydration
- Hepatocellular carcinoma

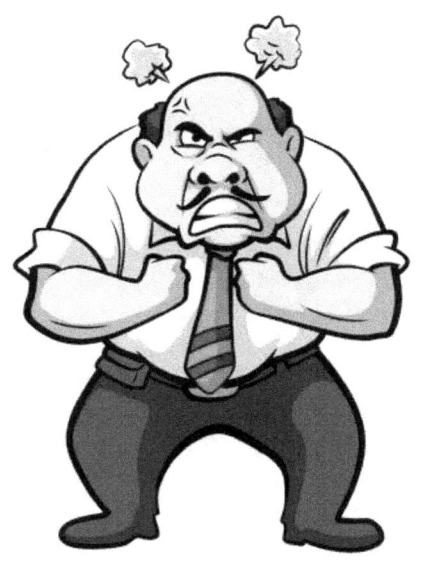

Hepatospenomegaly

CML gives Hepatosplenomegaly

. Myelofibrosis
. Lymphatic leukaemia
. Gaucher's disease
. Hairy cell leukaemia

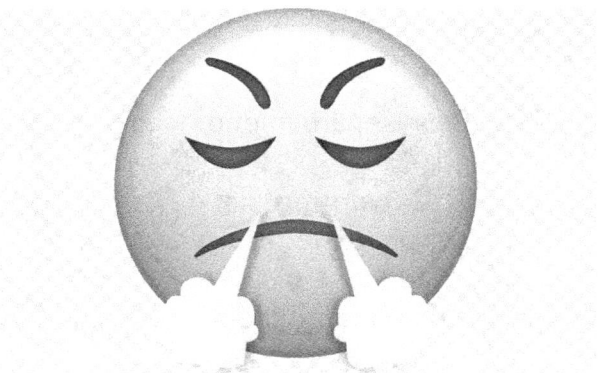

GI obstruction

Mnemonic: I Must Have a Shit Poo

- Inflammation
- Malignancy/Meckel's diverticulitis
- Hernia
- Adhesions

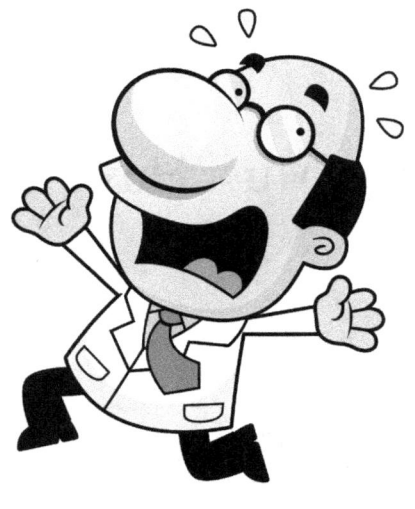

Hyperthyroidism

Mnemonic: Gave Too Much Thyroxine

. Grave's Disease
. Toxic Mulinodular goitre
. Toxic Adenoma

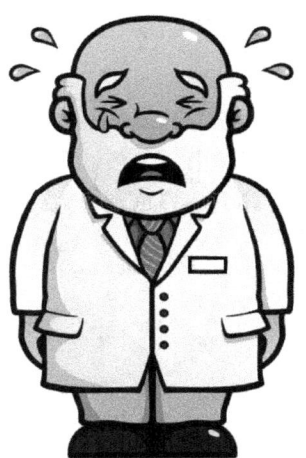

Osteomalacia

Mnemonic: 3L

. Low vitamin D
. Low calcium
. Low phosphate

Boo

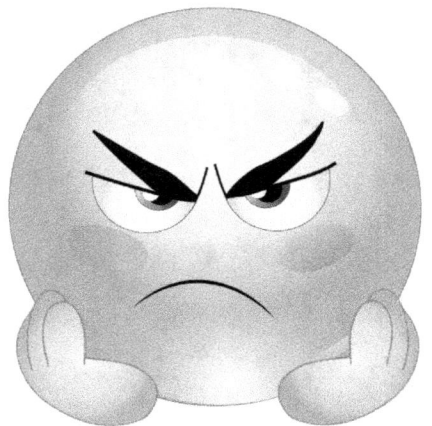

Polydipsia

Mnemonic: Patients keep drinking needlessly & constantly H2O (water)

. Primary polydipsia
. Kidney failure
. Dehydration/Diabetes/Drugs
. Nephrogenic diabetes insipidus
. Cranial diabetes insipidus
. Hypercalcemia

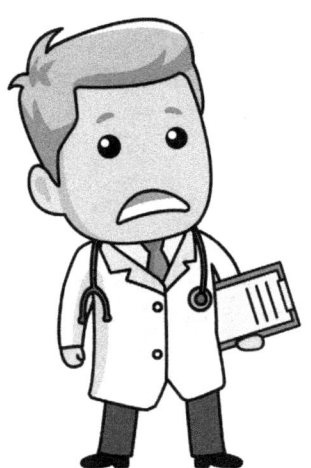

Prolactin level

6 Ps

. Pregnancy
. Polycystic ovary syndrome
. Prolactinoma
. Psychiatric drugs
. Primary hypothyroidism
. Pill

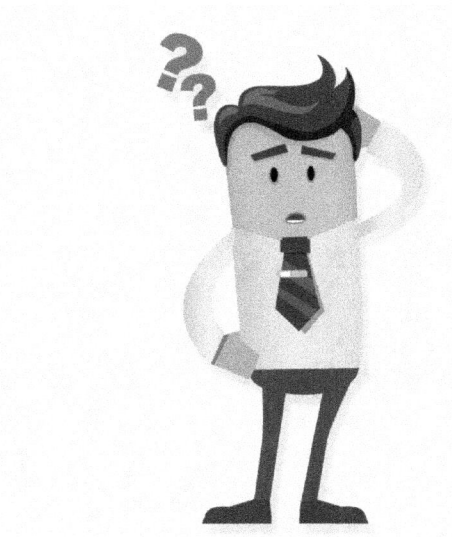

Nephritic syndrome

Hot Pee Output

. Haematuria /Hypertension
. Proteinuria
. Oedema/Oliguria

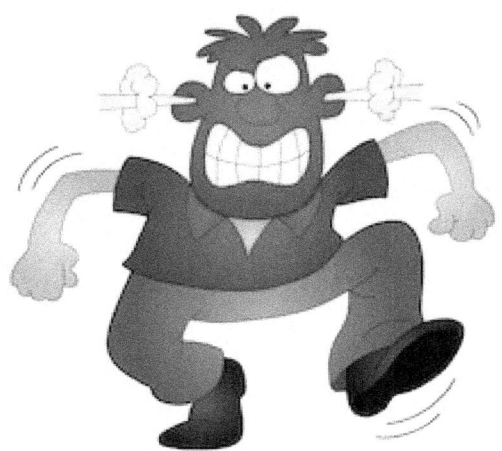

Acute Renal Failure

Intrinsic causes

Is Always Vasculitis & Glomerulonephritis

. Interstitial nephritis
. Acute tubular necrosis
. Vasculitis
. Glomerulonephritis

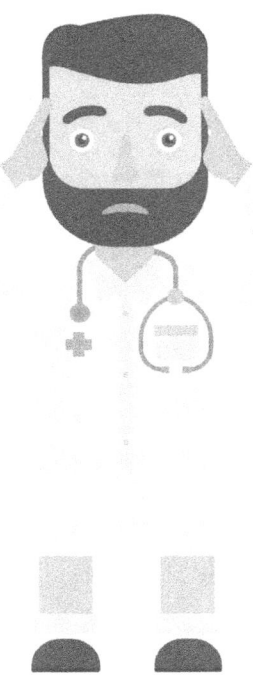

Collapsed Lung

POP Lung

- Pneumothorax
- Obstruction (foreign body, mucus)
- Pleural effusion
- Lymphadenopathy (cancer)

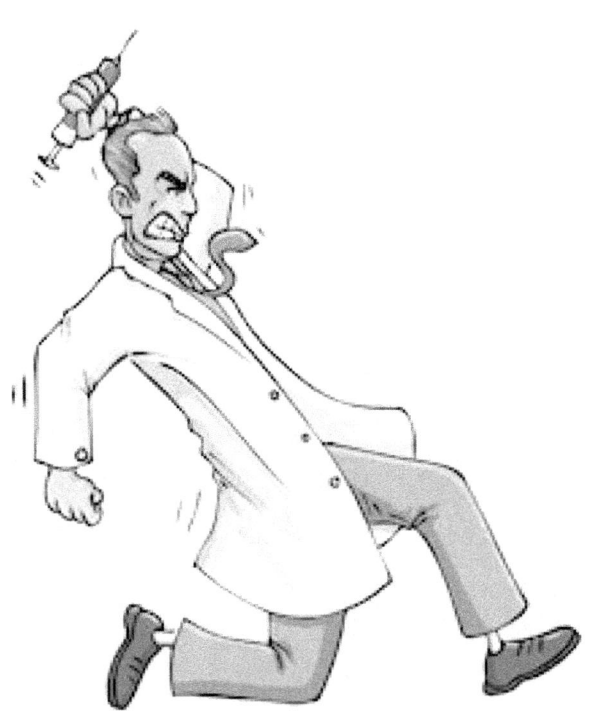

Cor Pulmonale

Emphysema Frequently Causes Cor Pulmonale

- Emboli
- Fibrosis
- COPD
- Primary pulmonary hypertension

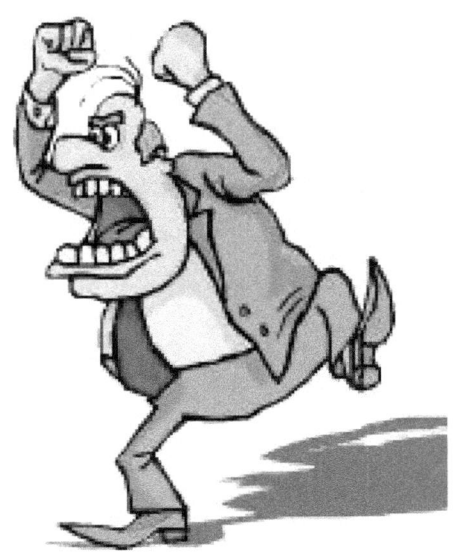

Empyema

Mnemonic: My Lung Secretes Pus & Black Shit

. Mediastinal sepsis
. Lung abscess
. Subphrenic abscess
. Pneumonia
. Bronchieactasis
. Surgery

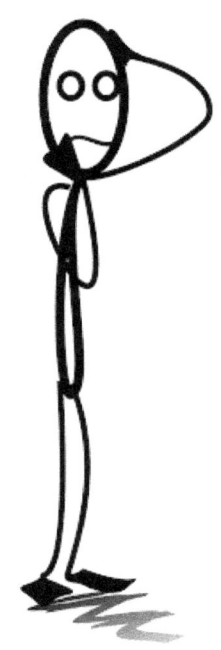

Haemoptysis

Mnemonic: Bloody Cough therefore LVF Maybe LVF

. Bronchieactasis
. Cancer
. Tuberculosis
. Mitral stenosis
. Left ventricular failure
. Pulmonary embolism/Pneumonia

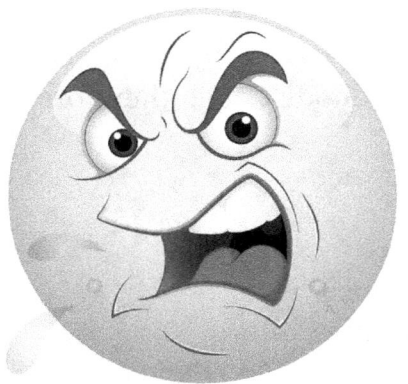

Pleural effusion

Exudate
Mnemonic: MR PISS

. Malignant effusion
. Rheumatoid arthritis
. Pulmonary embolism
. Infection
. SLE
. Subphrenic abscess

Transudate

Cardiac Liver Nephrotic

. Cardiac failure
. Liver failure
. Nephrotic syndrome

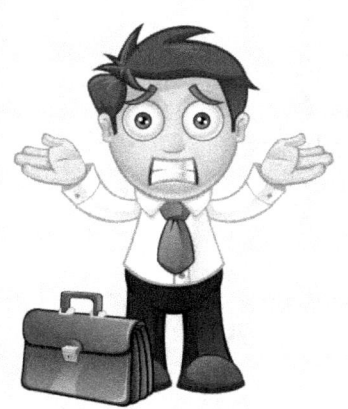

Pneumothorax

Please SIT

. Primary
. Secondary
. Iatrogenic
. Traumatic

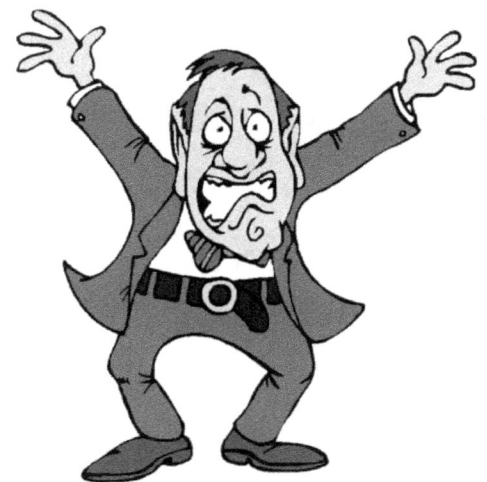

Upper lobe fibrosis

Mnemonic: BAD SCAR
- Bronchopulmonary Aspergillosis
- Allergic Alveolitis (EXtrinsic)
- Drugs (chemotherapy)
- Sarcoidosis
- Coal worker Pnemoconiosis
- Ankylosis spondylitis
- Radiation

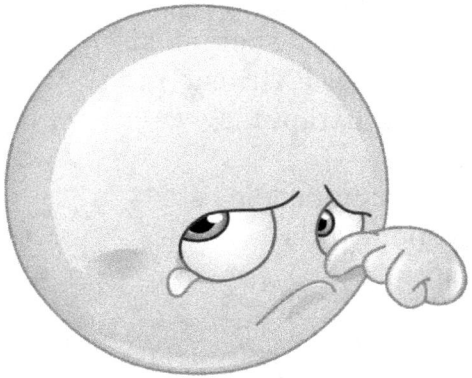

Monoarthrits

Mnemonic: Osteoarthritis gives severe pain

. Osteoarthritis
. Gout
. Septic arthritis
. Pseudo gout

www.ingramcontent.com/pod-product-compliance
Lightning Source LLC
Chambersburg PA
CBHW052345220526
45465CB00003BA/965